TELEMEDICINE

WHAT THE FUTURE HOLDS WHEN YOU'RE ILL

TELEMEDICINE

Maryann Karinch

New Horizon Press Far Hills, New Jersey

Requests for permission should be addressed to:
New Horizon Press
P.O. Box 669
Far Hills, NJ 07931

Karinch, Maryann.
Telemedicine: What the Future Holds When You're Ill

Library of Congress Catalog Card Number: 94-066757

ISBN: 0-88282-130-X (hc)
ISBN: 0-88282-131-8 (pb)

New Horizon Press

Manufactured in the U.S.A.

1998 1997 1996 1995 1994 / 5 4 3 2 1

To my mother, who heals from any distance

—M. K.

Table of Contents

Acknowledgments

This book was inspired by the United States Army, especially Lt. Col. Edward R. Gomez, who introduced me to the attempts made to bring the healing powers of Walter Reed Army Medical Center to Somalia and Croatia. I deeply appreciate the support that Ed gave me, as well as the Surgeon General of the Army, Alcide M. LaNoue, and many others, including: Lt. Col. Ron Poropatich, Col. Rick Satava, Maj. Gordy Murray, Sgt. Carl Boocks, Maj. J.B. Crowther, Lt. Col. Steve Broughall, Col. Fred Goeringer and his team at Fort Detrick, Col. Bill Wiessman, Maj. Tom Moore and the outstanding civilian members of the Walter Reed team, Fred Copeman and Dr. Linda Brink. Their gracious invitation to me to learn about their work and their genuine enthusiasm for telemedicine will always distinguish them.

I also heartily thank Dr. Jay Sanders at the Medical College of Georgia; Dr. Eric Tangalos; Marv Mitchell; Dr. Bijoy Khandheria; Dr. Robert Wood; John LaForgia at The Mayo Clinic; Jim Reid, who moved the Eastern Montana Telemedicine Network forward against many odds; Dr. Jane Preston, a truly dedicated and wise patron of telemedicine and founder of the American Telemedicine Association; the renowned surgeon Dr. Michael DeBakey; Dr. Max House, still controlling costs in Canada; Dr. Ace Allen, a champion of information sharing in the telemedicine community; Dr. Rashid Bashshur, whose standards originate from the mountaintop; Audun Rundhovde, a key figure in Norway's outstanding program; NASA's telemedicine-in-space team, Dr. Earl Ferguson, Dr. Don Stewart; and Chuck Doarn of Lockheed.

Important technical input also came from Paul Heller, the Army's consultant on telemedicine; Dr. Arthur Kaufman; Dr. Phil Green and Dr. Nachum Sacham at SRI; Greg Merril at High Techsplanations; inventor Hal Woodward; Ann Lasko-Harvill at New Leaf; Dr. Matthew T. Freedman at Georgetown University Medical Center; Jenny Fung at the Advanced Research Projects Agency; Michael Goldberger at MODA Systems; and many participants at the 1994 IMAGE Society conference and Spacebridge to Moscow.

I gratefully acknowledge the contributions of people who added to their work days by sharing valuable information and insights on a regular basis. The chief contributor is Steve Messere, an unbelievably good friend and smart person. I appreciate also the contributions of many others who kept me informed on current events, specifically Michael Gravino, Bill Adler, Lisa Swayne, Beth Dewey, Richard Willis, Joe Grenn, Rob Ufford, Ron Oklewicz, and Shannon Penberthy of the Health Industry Manufacturers Association.

My dear and intelligent friends Rick Graul, Dave Sanasack, Eileen Mengers and Jim Newman also contributed their opinions on style and content as the book developed. This help was valuable and deeply appreciated.

Lastly, thanks to my brother, who has always agreed with my mother and father that I can do anything.

Author's Note

This book is based on both my research and extensive interviews. In order to protect the identity of others, I have changed some people's names and identifying characteristics.

Introduction

Doctors are not gods, but technology can create the illusion that they are. Gods, by nature, are omniscient and omnipresent. Doctors, unfortunately, don't know everything and are bound by laws of time and distance no matter where they went to school or how fast they drive. Because even the most gifted medical professionals have natural limits, the role of technology in capturing, expanding and projecting what they know and what they do, is more than just titillating. Technology will shape the future of our health care.

The technology in question includes devices so small they could get lost in a drawer, so powerful that libraries of data can be searched and sorted in a heartbeat, and so capable of thrilling visual effects that Hollywood can't live without them. Hand-held computers with wireless communications; "smart cards" with everything about your medical history from conception to the present; miniature, remotely operated mechanical arms that cut, suction and sew; technology that creates computer-generated worlds—these are the examples of the technology of what we will call the "telemedicine revolution."

Telemedicine, broadly defined, is medicine that employs technology to deliver the best available health care anywhere, anytime. In isolated experiments, it has been practiced for decades. Now, telemedicine is starting to flourish, and the ramifications for worldwide health care are startling.

The following cases illustrate this point:

• In 1968, a medical school professor who was tired of wasting valuable time in Boston traffic initiated an interactive television project that allowed him to see emergency patients at Logan Airport in Boston without ever leaving Massachusetts General Hospital.

• In the mid-1980's, the Royal Flying Doctor Service used technology to conquer the vast distances that separated the inhabitants of many Queensland towns from good health care. The Australian government used a satellite network to bring doctors to thousands of remote Aborigines and Torres Strait Islanders.

• In 1993, the United States Army closed an 8,000-mile communication gap with a portable and inexpensive system that allowed doctors in Mogadishu, Somalia to get relatively quick help from specialists at the Walter Reed Army Medical Center. Pictures from a tent hospital allowed the physicians to ask a thousand questions, such as, "What kind of rash is this?" and "Why won't this wound heal?" Phone calls and faxes responded with diagnoses and treatment programs that saved lives and limbs.

• Lillehammer, Norway hosted more than the 1994 Winter Olympics. It was the site of a telecommunications project that linked the world's top surgeons to the small towns where athletes were taking high risks. Had there been a serious accident in a short-track skating event in Hamar or on the ice-hockey rink at Gjovik, these surgeons would be able to electronically have their eyes on the trauma. This should not strike us as strange, however. After all, every day of the Olympic Games, correspondents in Norway were engaged in real-time communication with their new anchors back home in New York, Tokyo or Rome. Why not have doctors do the same?

• In microengineering laboratories of the Swiss Federal Institute of Technology, researchers have developed an operation simulator. Capable of reproducing the natural resistance of the body organs in a virtual reality environment, doctors can practice a new surgery on it without using animals or cadavers.

In some of these cases, relatively simple communications and imaging technology was used to expand health care delivery systems. Another integral part of this digital world of medicine, however, is the highly sophisticated computer technology that enables innovations such as genetic engineering and the virtual reality surgical simulations done in Lausanne, Switzerland. This book explores the spectrum of technologies in the telemedicine revolution.

With a tip of the hat to history, this book explores the exciting futuristic concept of telemedicine of today and tomorrow with a deliberate emphasis on programs and projects that appear grounded in, and guided by, a scientific or methodical approach to upgrading health care delivery systems. The application of technology to realize the goal of universal access to high-quality medicine has been taking shape for decades. We should nurture, but not stifle, this movement through commitment to performance and technical standards.

Extraordinary innovations that will benefit the whole world emerge from that commitment on a regular basis. Some advanced technologies covered in this book have received developmental support from the United States Defense Department and/or from the National Aeronautics and Space Administration (NASA). Others have received support from Russian agencies as well as several European countries.

NASA and its sister space agencies around the world have a profound role in medical progress. More than serving as the agents for satellite communication among medical professionals, they also routinely support in-flight bioscience and health care research. After all, space agencies such as NASA are charged with providing care to the most remote people—those in space—so they must develop and sustain expertise in telemedicine.

Included in current and future technology on land and in space are incredible developments such as telepresence surgery, which is surgery performed by a distant physician with the help of a robotic arm, and internal physical examinations using tiny robots. In this world of next-generation tools, emergency medical technicians and nurses will resuscitate and operate under the guidance of a surgeon miles away. As optimistic as this sounds, issues linked to liability, fees and record keeping are among those that could slow telemedicine's progress in many countries.

There also are the financial, ethical and legal debates affecting the implementation of telemedicine which must be considered. So, while dramatic stories of telemedicine in action underline need, and glimpses of medicine in the near future inspire hope, it would be foolish to imply that there are no big impediments on the road to progress. Included in these considerations are sorting faulty objections from legitimate concerns for patient privacy and welfare.

Telemedicine

Telemedicine puts medical resources exactly where they need to be—near the patient. It's a logical and normal application of communications, imaging and computer technology. Telemedicine, practiced with the same high standards to which we hope all medicine aspires, should be a fundamental element of health care improvement and reform worldwide.

No matter how revolutionary the advances of high technology medicine are, however, no one should forget the ever present need in patient care for a gentle, human touch. The day a doctor uses interactive television to announce, "Mr. Jones, you have six days to live," is the day someone should cut that doctor's cables.

To sum it up, "Star Trek" medicine is not some science fiction creation of the future, it has already begun in the present. From genetic engineering to robot surgeons, from liquid breathing for premature babies to computer programming of injured spinal cords, new technology in the medical environment is helping mere mortals perform miracles.

A miracle is supposed to be something beyond our comprehension, beyond our ability to duplicate at will. The concept conjures up images of singular events never to be repeated, the crutches of the cured hanging by the grotto at Lourdes, or Moses parting the Red Sea with a staff. Yet these are not the only kind of miracles. The far-reaching and creative, inspired application of new technology in the medical environment adds another definition. The new meaning of the word "miracle" is an awe-inspiring feat that can be precisely duplicated over and over again for the benefit of each one of us.

1

A Glimpse of What the Future Holds

The twenty-first century will be information-based. Initially, this will only be a minor trend, but by the middle of the twenty-first century, it will dominate our approach to health care delivery. The key technologies to this change will be telecommuting, teleconferencing, teleconsultation, and telesurgery.

Joseph M. Rosen, MD
Department of Plastic & Reconstructive Surgery
Dartmouth Hitchcock Medical Center

One of the most profound of telemedicine's new models in health care is bringing the doctor to the patient, like an old-fashioned house call. This switch from a doctor-based to a patient-based health care system is at the heart of telemedicine.

This may sound like fantasy, but it is really a logical outcome of the world going digital. The first stage in this process featured room-sized computers that centralized data processing. Gaining access to it was like using many modern medical facilities, requiring getting in the car, driving to the location, parking, walking down the hall, filling out paperwork, then standing in line. Steadily, technological advances transformed those early behemoths into an individual tool, a *personal* computer.

Telemedicine's new, breakthrough technological advances can help health care move in the same direction. With them, patients around the world, many in third world countries or backwoods areas, can get more specialized—as well as more personalized—care. Patients can sometimes literally access the skill of medical experts, on-demand and in the home. Providing the best care—anywhere—is what telemedicine is all about.

Some of the new technology covered in this book already exists in medical centers and corporate, military and university labs. Some are even sold in a few stores. Others will be available in the near future. With such innovative health care becoming available, but as not yet widely disseminated, there are questions each of us who may need this care should ask. Among them are:

What does this revolution in health care mean if you have a brain tumor, breast cancer, malaria or an arthritic hip? What does it mean if you live in a remote Russian village shaken by an earthquake or on a frozen spit on the most remote edge of Canada? What does it mean if you are wounded on a battlefield or hit by a truck on a country road? These questions lead to true stories of medical miracles.

In a 1994 video tape, former United States Surgeon General C. Everett Koop told the United States Congress and White House staff about telemedicine and the trend toward using it for patient-based health care. In that tape, he tells the story of a 79-year-old New England farmer named Joe. Joe has had a small freckle on his face for 15 years; now it's growing. Joe is afraid it's cancer and that it could pose a serious threat to his health. Joe had a stroke last year, suffers from diabetes and doesn't drive anymore, so a trip to a specialist fifty miles away would be a real burden. His wife goes with him to the neighborhood doctor, who notices there are dark spots inside the large freckle. "I'm just not sure how important that is," she says. "I'd like to bring in Dr. Spencer, a dermatologist I've worked with in the past." Joe balks at the thought of the long drive. When the doctor explains that she has arranged for the specialist to join them in her office and has already sent preliminary photos and material, Joe is amazed. The doctor points to what looks like a television set.

With the push of a button, a life-size image of the dermatologist appears on the screen and the consultation begins. In telling Joe how his freckle has changed since photos were last taken two years ago, the distant specialist activates a cube-shaped monitor. The monitor, which sits in the family doctor's office, has displays on all sides. Joe, his wife across the room, and both physicians see the same images at the same time. The dermatologist explains that a biopsy must be performed on the freckle. He also puts on the monitor statistics about skin cancer to emphasize that Joe must use sun screen. The family doctor tells Joe that she will talk with him again after she gets the results of the test.

A couple of days later, the pathologist who performed the biopsy electronically, joins the dermatologist and family doctor in their respective offices for a quick meeting. The three-dimensional monitor allows the pathologist to display a diagram indicating to what level of tissue the cancer has progressed. For the dermatologist, the required excision would present no problem, but to the family practitioner who has never removed anything this large from this part of the face, the procedure poses a formidable challenge. The dermatologist maps out the surgery on a computer-generated head displayed on the monitor. The cube-shaped monitor actually conveys a three-dimensional perspective. With the surgical instructions complete, the family practitioner downloads the information to her desktop computer so she can review the surgery and practice the procedure through simulation. The surgery is successful and Joe gets well.

The northeastern United States is not the only spot on the globe where patient-based medicine is taking shape, however. Joe could have just as easily been a fisherman in a Newfoundland village or a sheep herder in Norway. All over the world, major medical centers are using technology to bridge the distant gap between urban physicians and rural patients.

Primarily, Koop's story asserts that the technology will profoundly affect to what degree health care will become personalized and specialized because of telemedicine. The nature of medical record keeping, the physical examination, surgery, health maintenance and health education will change out of necessity. And the technology to do all of it is at hand.

To start, every individual will need to be tied informationally to a health care system. This may be compared to the widespread and growing use of automated teller machines (ATMs). The convenience and advantages of being tied informationally to a financial system 24 hours a day, seven days a week, in numerous parts of the world are tremendous. The convenience and advantages for a doctor gaining access to a person's health records are even more outstanding.

One tool for accomplishing this might be the so-called "smart card," originally conceived of as bank of card-sized devices that store data on an embedded microprocessor or "chip." They would give quick access to a few critical facts about the owner such as whether he or she is classified as "diabetic," "asthmatic," "schizophrenic." Prototypes made in the early 1990's stored about a page of text information and featured a thumb-sized photograph pasted on the front to increase the card's value as an identification tool. This model was woefully inadequate, however. To ensure its value as a health care device, the card would have to be a true digital device containing such detailed data as a picture, signature, perhaps a fingerprint or eye scan, pharmaceutical information, allergies and immunizations, dental records, a basic description of all surgeries and any other relevant information.

All of this can be accomplished with new approaches to compressing or squeezing information to alter dramatically the functional range of such a device. "Meditag" is an example of a system that has so much memory that it can store more than basic medical data. Depending on the region or country, a multiple-use tag could store military service records, academic and employment histories, or social welfare payments. It could also contain information about a genetic predisposition to alcoholism, Huntington's disease or cancer—a fact that immediately raises issues of privacy and confidentiality.

What if it were possible for a thief, or just the wrong person, to read the volumes of private information stored on a smart card? The developers, Lloyd "Hal" Woodward and Arthur Kaufman, partially addressed this aspect of the privacy/confidentiality issue by designing a two-tag system meant to be used with any computer. The ward or emergency room clerk in a hospital would dock an incoming patient's tag, as well as the clerk's "access tag," in ports externally mounted on a computer. Access to limited information would enable the clerk to process the patient more quickly, thereby facilitating treatment. The emergency room physician would have access privileges for a wider range of medical data, as would the person's family doctor. The information on the card flows back and forth, the ports on the tag connect with ports on the computer and infrared light transmits signals between them.

A corollary benefit to such a system is automatic creation of a "paper trail." When the physician inserts the two tags, this action is logged, so that a record of who examined the patient, and why thy did so, become embedded on the tag.

This model presents other advantages, too. First, it eliminates the scratching and demagnetizing concerns associated with smart cards designed like bank cards, that is, with a magnetic strip on the back. Second, the embedded identification information includes personal images, rendering it rather pointless to steal.

Still other questions arise, however. What if it gets lost? To be more realistic, what happens *when* it gets lost? If that's true, perhaps the best solution is to store a "master copy" of the information on a chip inside our bodies. Embedding critical data, similar to storing flight information on the black box in an aircraft, could ensure the existence of a personal record, as well as yield quick answers in a post-mortem examination. In addition, just as the bank manages to update records as transactions are made, a health care system could do the same with at least a portion of the personal data.

Given that the individual's records will appear on some kind of tag or card, the waiting room exercise of filling out a history form will be eliminated. The patient can proceed straight to a physical exam, knowing that key images and text are at the doctor's disposal. This kind of database of medical information was illustrated in Koop's story about Joe. One thing the story didn't cover, however, is that Joe's health could be monitored every day without him ever leaving home.

In Fall 1994, the Medical College of Georgia (MCG) set a precedent in telemedicine worldwide by establishing test sites for home health care systems. They were installed in twenty-five homes of people with chronic conditions who were constantly being readmitted to the hospital—so-called "revolving door patients." The unidirectional cable that brought MTV, home shopping and CNN into their homes was modified to deliver interactive capability.

By monitoring patients at home, health care providers should be able to avert trips to the emergency room and admission to the hospital. Depending on the patient's need, the remote monitoring devices in the "smart box" on the television set or computer monitor could include an EKG, stethoscope, digital blood pressure cuff and pulse meter, pulse oximeter to measure blood oxygen level, peak expiratory flow rate meter to allow for pulmonary function studies and a blood chemistry analysis device. Since Joe was a stroke victim with diabetes, he might have the deluxe model at his house.

Sounds expensive, doesn't it? Even at the highest cost of about $10,000 per system, the MCG prototype is decidedly cost-effective. Here are two examples of how it could avert emergencies:

Carol, an asthmatic patient, is experiencing increased airway resistance. This phenomenon occurs weeks before respiratory failure and can be treated if identified promptly. The monitoring system would detect this problem, and the patient would not abruptly find herself in the intensive care unit some night.

Gerald, a patient with congestive heart failure, starts to gain weight. If the small physiological changes that occur with that weight gain are detected and the trend is reversed promptly, he will not end up in the emergency room two weeks later with pulmonary edema.

On the basis of current rates in the United States, each one of these patients will incur bills of $15,000 to $25,000 for a short hospital stay, while the home system will cost only a fraction as much.

MCG's next home system will even more closely mimic a house call: *The distant doctor will also be able to touch the patient.*

Until the newer virtual-reality technologies had been developed, the thought of a remote physician touching or palpating a patient over a telemedicine network was material only for science fiction. Now, through adaptation by the Georgia Institute of Technology of a virtual reality tool called a DataGlove, doctors at MCG will be able to use an electronic hand to feel the texture, shape and temperature of a distant patient's body. The hand will reproduce the sensation of an object under the skin. For example, a doctor could detect an enlarged liver by feeling the person's abdomen.

Even more exciting is the news that the techniques now being practiced merely hint at the possible technicolor wonders of telemedicine.

2

Uptown Medicine on the Network

We have the opportunity here in Washington, at Walter Reed, as you do in Moscow, to walk between floors or parts of the hospital to see different specialists. But it's through mechanisms such as the Spacebridge and other telemedicine initiatives that we can all bring to bear the specialty expertise in our medical centers at remote sites.

Maj. Yancy Phillips, MD
Walter Reed Army Medical Center

Because of new innovations, specialists and subspecialists from around the world roam hospital corridors, chatting about new forms of spinal membrane repair or about surgery on a valve in the left ventricle of the heart. Stories of amazing cures and impossible surgeries emanate from those corridors. Unfortunately, ready access to that level of expertise is rare. Most people in North America and in the countries of Europe, the Middle East and the Far East are lucky to receive basic care in times of illness and injury.

Telemedicine will radically change that fact. It will mean universal access to quality health care by making the practice of medicine more independent of time and distance constraints. It means using technology to put the keenest medical minds and sharpest surgical skills where they belong—with the patient, no matter where that person is.

The future of health care is inextricably linked to telemedicine, and by looking at how telemedicine is evolving today, we can get a real glimpse of what tomorrow holds for both the able-bodied and the seriously ill.

The CAT scan indicated a tumor in the liver, on the lower portion near the gall bladder. As a result of a long-standing hepatitis infection, advanced liver cirrhosis had set in; Henry Rodriguez, the patient, was a prime candidate for liver cancer. To get another look at the problem, Dr. Joseph M. Collins used ultrasound, which uses sound waves to generate a picture. With the ultrasound probe in his left hand and the biopsy needle in his right, he set out to assess whether or not the mass was malignant.

With his fears confirmed, Collins faced having to tell the patient that he had an aggressive form of cancer that would kill him in about one year if left unchecked. Surgery was out because Rodriguez also suffered from severe heart disease, among other things. He probably wouldn't have survived an operation. Chemotherapy and radiation therapy have little effect on this type of cancer, so Collins discarded those options as well. He searched for another answer. It was 1990; medical literature of the time talked about a new technique in which alcohol injections were used to ablate liver tumors.

Dr. Collins made a call from his hospital, the Mayo Clinic in Scottsdale, Arizona. He called Dr. William Charboneau who had used the technique at the Mayo Clinic in Rochester, Minnesota. Both of the doctors were subspecialists in their field, specifically, diagnostic and interventional radiology. They agreed that the location and size of the patient's cancer made him a prime candidate for the alcohol therapy. Unfortunately, the patient was too sick to travel to Rochester. They decided that Charboneau would guide Collins through the procedure over an interactive video conference link the following Monday.

The procedure was to be a minor exercise for the patient, who could remain awake, but a trial by fire for Collins. As the two doctors and their patient observed the initial ultrasound images together, 1,000 miles apart, Collins measured the tumor. On the bottom of the satellite picture, Charboneau could see the result: 40.8 millimeters (mm) was the current diameter of the cancer. It had grown 8 mm in the past week. From this baseline, they would be able to gauge their progress and success. During the critical moments of the procedure, their conversation went as follows:

Dr. Charboneau: ". . . I'd probably use that (route for the needle) as a second choice and the transverse as a first choice, because that view is pretty straightforward. Lots of room to watch the needle come down, so if you slide the transducer a little to the left, toward the top, and then imagine coming down, you'll want to—yeah, that right there would be a very doable position. Almost straight down. A little bit angled in."

Dr. Collins: "Almost like along the edge of the view here."

Charboneau: "Yeah, but I would probably have the whole thing in the field of view, or almost the whole thing—go down a little bit, right about there. Yeah. You know, that's certainly a doable position, too. If you're comfortable with that, you know,

I would do that, too. That's nice. Take it to the back. Beautiful. That's just where you want to be. Now I'd start with a picture there. OK, have him take a breath in."

Collins: "Take a breath in, Mr. Rodriguez. Hold your breath."

Charboneau: "Get your best view. There you go. Now go ahead, give it a blast."

Collins: "Now breathe, Mr. Rodriguez. Another breath in, Mr. Rodriguez. Hold your breath."

Charboneau: "You'll see the tip there . . . push it forward just a snitch and give it another little blast while you got a good view. There you go. Not too much further forward."

Collins: "Another deep breath in, Mr. Rodriguez. Hold your breath."

Charboneau: "Perfect. Perfect."

After another blast, Charboneau confirmed: "I think you've done it! Incredible job, you did great!" Patient follow-up would involve another interactive video link in two days. The CAT scans taken after the procedure showed that the tumor had been completely removed. The patient remained cancer-free until his death three years later from heart disease.

This case is a stunning example of how telemedicine can bring the best new treatment to a patient in a distant location. As a corollary, the scene demonstrates how physicians can engage in telementoring, or coaching at a distance.

The recently built, marble Mayo Building at the heart of the main complex has nineteen floors. Gargoyles ring the upper floors of its predecessor across the street, a classic structure crowned by a bell tower. Within the building is an integrated practice of people who care for patients, conduct research and teach.

A goliath in the medical community for many reasons, those who guide it have great financial resources, business acumen and a professional desire to sustain a customized telemedicine network that relies on satellites. Whereas the terms "off-the-shelf" and "telephone lines" imply some kind of cost constraints in a telemedicine network, "customized" and "satellite" do not.

With the mutually supportive aims of preserving the Mayo culture and expanding its excellence in health care delivery, the mother clinic ensured that its satellite offspring in Jacksonville, Florida and Scottsdale, Arizona were born into a communications network with interactive video capability. This gave doctors at all sites the capability to build camaraderie and exchange ideas; it also gave the powers-that-be in Rochester the ability, literally, to keep an eye on things in the field.

At the time this network was established, with the Jacksonville clinic opening in October 1986 and Scottsdale the following June, many other telemedicine programs around the world had either died of financial starvation or not yet been launched. It would be wrong to say that Mayo "set the pace" or "showed others the way," however. Mayo's system is different, supporting the extremely high-level imagery and communications requirements of subspecialists, like Dr. Collins and Dr. Charboneau.

Canadian specialists, facing cost constraints, chose another route. Memorial University of Newfoundland (MUN) in St. John's sits on the piece of Canada's far-eastern province that juts into the icy Atlantic. It helps serve the health care and health education needs of 600,000 people scattered over a large area.

One morning, a six-year-old boy in Labrador City, which is separated from St. John's by a strait and hundreds of miles of rough terrain, had an epileptic seizure. The family panicked. They rushed the child to the local hospital, where their family doctor met them. The doctor was confused and concerned—this child had never before shown signs of the disorder. Immediately, he turned to the specialists at MUN, which has operated a telemedicine system since 1977. Using facsimile equipment like that found in offices around the world, the doctor transmitted the child's EEG (electroencephalogram) to the hospital at St. John's. Within an hour, the response came back. The family physician told the anxious parents that their son had a benign form of epilepsy that could easily be controlled with medication. There was no brain damage and no need to airlift the boy to a pediatrician at MUN. Their panic and the emergency was over.

3

Technology Catches up with Need

What is important here is that telemedicine is a system without borders. It is not a new kind of medicine. It is a way of communication that makes it possible to utilize existing medical resources in a new and much more efficient way.

Steinar Pedersen, MD
Head of the Department of Telemedicine
University Hospital of Tromsoe, Norway

Tombstones of past decades recorded many deaths a doctor could have prevented easily, but in those times, the doctor was fifty or more miles away. When the telephone gained popularity, physicians tried to close the geographic gap by responding to those callers had minor complaints with advice: "Sounds like a migraine. Take two aspirin . . ."

These phone calls were the earliest, simplest practice of telemedicine. As technology evolved and the problems because of distant patients grew, it drove telemedicine toward greater functionality. At first, the doctor could just hear the distant patient or colleague. The next step was sight—actually transmitting images to determine diagnosis and treatment.

Ken Bird hated sitting in traffic on his way from to Boston's Logan Airport medical station, where he served as the first director. Designed to provide emergency services for passengers, the clinic opened after an unnecessarily tragic collision in 1962 between a prop-jet and a flock of birds on the runway. During that incident, gawking crowds prevented emergency vehicles from reaching many of the victims in time. As a result, many of them drowned in shallow water.

Early in the medical station operation, some nurses called Bird to report that an older woman had badly injured herself in a fall. They didn't want to move her without guidance from a doctor. He had to get in the car and drive out there, but the thought occurred to him that there must be a way he could "see" the patient from Massachusetts General—a way he could watch her on television, like the "Ed Sullivan Show." Thirty feet under the Charles River, in the tunnel that joins Boston to Logan, he developed a plan for "telediagnosis." This vision would make Kenneth T. Bird the first big name in telemedicine.

"I thought it was the craziest idea I'd ever heard," recalls Dr. Jay H. Sanders, a resident at Mass General at the time, when he heard Bird's concept. Sanders was among those who watched Bird configure a two-way television system under a grant from the United States Public Health Service. Bird planned to combine television monitors with microwave units to transmit signals, thereby creating a full-motion interactive video service. Then bureaucracy stepped in. He couldn't find microwave channels acceptable to the Federal Communications

Commission (FCC), so the FCC delayed giving permission to activate the link until April 1968.

The first patient to benefit from the project had an acutely swollen left knee. The nurse at the Logan medical station positioned the camera and conducted an examination in full view of the physician at Mass General. The doctor then made the correct diagnosis: an acute traumatic intrapatella bursitis. Over television, doctor and patient discussed the treatment and medication was prescribed. As Bird tells the story in a 1975 paper delivered at a physicians' conference at the University of Michigan, when the patient prepared to leave he was asked, "Well, sir, what do you think of this?" He reportedly responded, "Why, doc, it's just as if you were here."

When physicians at Mass General and the medical assistants at the airport facility were finally able to have eye-to-eye contact, the latter assumed an expanded role as a clinic for area residents and airport employees.

Bird and his colleagues at Massachusetts General tested the system's reliability by comparing remote diagnoses with those done on the same patients in face-to-face visits. The tests yielded impressive results: when the two diagnoses were compared, a striking 98 percent of those done over the crude interactive television system were accurate. The remaining 2 percent might be better characterized as "over-protective," rather than wrong. In other words, if the physician diagnosing over the system was not certain, he or she tended to err on the conservative side to protect the patient.

In that same 1975 article in which Bird threw the spotlight on this new thing called "telemedicine," he confidently declared: "Microwave transmission and interpretation of electrocardiograms [EKGs] and roentgenograms [X-rays] is as accurate as direct visualization. Stethoscopy [use of a stethoscope to hear the heart] and microscopy are also accurately performed and interpreted via the system."

The issue of whether or not patients would respond well to the camera received a critical look from Mass General's psychiatry department. When the system was set up, all the medical chiefs of service embraced it except for one—Dr. Tom Dwyer, Chief of Psychiatry. Sanders recalls that Dwyer "would stick his head in the door of the telemedicine room at least once a week. Then he would close the door and walk down the hall. As he walked away, shaking his head in disgust, he'd say, 'This will never work in psychiatry.'" Dwyer told Ken Bird he would never be able to reproduce with cold technology the special feeling of warmth and ambiance that is required to exist between a psychiatrist and his or her patient.

But Bird was a maverick. Rather than argue, he secured additional funding and set up a second satellite site at the New Bedford Veterans Administration Psychiatric Hospital, which was a facility that faculty from Mass General would visit daily to see patients. Three years after they launched this study of "telepsychiatry," the clinicians at New Bedford wrote a series of papers on the incredible effectiveness of the new process. They found that, not only could they achieve the desired ambience, they could also manipulate it. They discovered what any television or film director could have told them in a minute about frame tension—that the emotions of a scene are shaped not merely by the dialogue or facial expression, but also by the way the scene is shot. The psychiatrists found that, when they got to a particular point that needed emphasis, they could move to a close-up. As the patient watched the screen, the doctor's face would begin to fill it, leaving the impression that the words were coming from a higher authority. Conversely, when the psychiatrist found a point which was too sensitive for the patient to deal with comfortably, the camera could pull away, thereby reducing the intensity of the moment by miniaturizing the psychiatrist in the background. Soon, the patients insisted on having the ability to control the size of the doctor's face. The system was altered to allow for it this, granting psychiatric patients greater control over their treatment.

From 1973 to 1976, while at the University of Miami, Sanders studied the psychological impact of this early form of telemedicine on many kinds of patients, not just psychiatric ones. Under a $1.2 million National Science Foundation Grant, this study was one aspect of a major investigation that also covered the quality, economics and technology of the telemedicine project. He and his co-investigators found that doctors and patients alike were drawn to the camera, lured the same way shoppers in an electronics store are to a monitor that shows them walking by. Almost everyone liked being on television, and within a few minutes of their experience, a natural conversation blossomed. It was reassuring to telemedicine's pioneers to see patients feel so comfortable with the technology that they could tell the intimate details of their life to a doctor not physically present.

Bird tried to alert colleagues to the long-term implications of applying communications and cameras to the practice of medicine. He could see that the biggest problem worldwide—just making sure that people had access to care—could be chipped away with telemedicine. In his 1975 presentation, he even tried to awaken practical sensibilities in his audience by underlining telemedicine's cost-effective nature:

The cost of building one mile of a four-lane highway in non-urban, semirural, or rural Massachusetts is four million dollars. If one paid reasonable value on the property which is acquired to build this one mile highway, it would cost another one million dollars. To create two telemedicine centers from twenty to forty miles apart, the current total cost is about seventy-thousand dollars. In short, a modest expenditure of funds for capital investment would allow the medicine of today to become "airborne."

Jay Sanders continued preaching telemedicine after his work at Mass General ceased, but it was not until many years later that he fully resumed his pioneering work in telemedicine by establishing a robust program based at the Medical College of Georgia. Shortly thereafter, as telemedicine became a talked-about concept among doctors all over the world, Kenneth T. Bird, whom many consider the father of telemedicine, died.

In Canada, while the Mass General project withered from lack of funds, Dr. A. Max House joined Bird in the history books. At the Memorial University of Newfoundland (MUN) in St. John's, he set up what is now the oldest continually operating telemedicine program in the world.

In preparation for launching a telemedicine experiment with the Canadian Space Program in 1977, Dr. House studied a sampling of early efforts: Mass General, NASA's work beaming medical expertise to Native American reservations, and a full-motion television consulting facility linking Ponce, the lone major city on Puerto Rico's Caribbean side, with a town 110 miles away. House took a different path, though. Using the joint Canada/United States Hermes Satellite, he opted for a *one*-way television/two-way interactive audio configuration. For a three-month trial period, four remote hospitals were linked to the University in St. John's.

At the end of the trial, project coordinators began to have second thoughts. Certainly, they had demonstrated the value of television in piping medical education and expertise to remote doctors, but they had to admit they could have done the same thing at a much lower cost with simpler technology. Their redirected efforts launched a terrestrially-based teleconference system established in 1979 that is still in existence today.

On June 14, 1994 Max House wrote about the endurance of his system:

> In the early days, people were very keen on glamorous television projects. Back in the late seventies and early eighties, they found that while the projects could be supported, at the end of the project there was no money to continue with an operational system. It was because we chose to not do the expensive projects, and concentrated on relatively inexpensive audio and audio-plus projects, that we were able to build up a system that functioned over the years and modestly grew. It gave us experience, so that when the technology evolved, we were able to take advantage of it. Now we have the best of all worlds.

In the mid-eighties, House went on to make more history by stretching out to Africa and the Caribbean. In 1985, the International Satellite Organization (Intelsat) and the International Institute of Communications established the Satellites in Health and Rural Education (SHARE) project to celebrate Intelsat's twentieth birthday. At the time, MUN pediatricians had special ties to the Pediatric Department at Makerere University in Kampala, Uganda, to which they provided counsel through support from the Canadian International Development Agency.

The Telemedicine Group at MUN gave a new dimension to the interaction by using the SHARE project to set up a telemedicine link. This network involved teleconferencing between facilities in Nairobi, Kenya, and Kampala, with a link from those two East African cities to MUN. During the ten-month life of the project that began in February 1986, roughly 100 EEGs were transmitted from East Africa to the MUN staff. Intelsat charged nothing for the satellite facilities. Equipment at the remote site featured an electrode cap and transmitter. The latter converted brain wave patterns to analog signals in the voice bandwidth for transmission over the network. In other words, the brain wave patterns became like words in an ordinary conversation over phone lines.

MUN took the SHARE project another step in June 1986 by reaching out to six Caribbean countries on the University of the West Indies teleconference system. Although terminated a mere 6 months later, the experiment did form the foundation for a successful data and voice transmission venture called the Intra-Jamaican project.

4

Spacebridge: Telemedicine Between Nations

Today we can earnestly talk about the birth of telemedicine in my country. You have become part of our future in this work.

Ashot Sarkisian, MD
Co-chair of the Spacebridge to Moscow
Summary Session, June 24, 1994

After Canada used telemedicine in Africa and the Caribbean, other dramatic demonstrations of this technology's international capabilities followed. The first such demonstration occurred in the wake of the massive earthquake which crumbled Soviet Armenia. On December 7, 1988, a few seconds of violent trembling caused 25,000 deaths. Another 125,000 victims of the devastation suffered head and spinal injuries, crushed limbs and organs, loss of blood, and disfiguring wounds. Armenia's medical system was crippled. Many health care workers were among the dead.

Doctors from all the republics of the Soviet Union rushed to the scene, but the range of injuries and the sheer number of victims overwhelmed them. Two weeks after the tragedy, NASA proposed to the Soviet Government that the two nations could activate a satellite-based medical consultation network. The goal was to transmit expertise to Soviet medical personnel in areas where they had an expressed need, namely, in plastic and reconstructive surgery, physical and psychological rehabilitation, public health and epidemiology. In NASA's vision, the link could come under the auspices of the existing bilateral Space Agreement between the United States and the Soviet Union Concerning the Exploration and Use of Outer Space for Peaceful Purposes.

Called "Telemedicine Spacebridge," the project got tangled, but not strangled, in paperwork in both countries. The idea for telemedicine consultations was a simple one. The implementation was a maze of procedural and technical questions. When would consultations occur? Who would handle translations? How would the transmissions be encrypted to protect the privacy of patients? Teams from both countries had to develop new standards for medical information transmission, as well as protocols and schedules on conducting the consultations.

Deeper questions lay at the heart of the delay, however. The Americans wanted to know what the Soviet doctors faced on a daily basis. The Soviets wanted to know how the American hospitals were different from theirs. In March, the American team traveled to Spitak, the largest city near the earthquake epicenter, to get a first-hand look at the destruction. They visited the Yerevan Republic Diagnostic Center to meet their Soviet counterparts and to see the rooms in which they worked and the instruments they used. A reciprocal trip by the Soviets to American sites followed in April. Meanwhile, NASA was constructing a web of communications among four major

United States hospitals on the Spacebridge.

Finally, five months after the tremors stopped, American and Soviet physicians opened a steady dialogue over a one-way video, two-way audio link. On May 4, 1989, they began tackling the post-acute rehabilitative needs of Armenia's sick and injured, and the slow process of rebuilding Armenia's medical system.

Broadcasts ran Monday through Friday, from 6 P.M. to 10 P.M. Armenian time (9 A.M. to 1 P.M. U.S. Eastern Daylight Time). Every Friday, Armenian doctors faxed patient information for the following week's discussions to medical personnel in the United States. The following Monday, the Americans would fax their Armenian colleagues journal articles and papers relevant to the cases. On Tuesday, Wednesday and Thursday, the cases were presented with the Soviet physicians examining patients in front of the camera and transmitting X-rays, CAT scans and ultrasound images. Despite some problems, the Spacebridge clearly moved patient care forward and marked the beginning of a new age of international cooperation.

Then, tragedy struck again on June 4, 1989, near the town of Ufa in Northern Russia. Two trains passed each other in a cloud of natural gas which was leaking from a pipeline. The gas sparked an explosion which killed hundreds of people and caused a thousand more to suffer burns and trauma. One of the trains was carrying mostly children.

This time, with the telemedicine link already in place, American physicians were able to aid their Soviet counterparts in the heat of the emergency. Quick cooperation between Soviet and American officials put a satellite station at the Ufa Medical Center. Connected by ground links to Yerevan, it was serviced by both the American and Armenian medical specialists.

By July 28, when the Spacebridge officially ended, 210 cases had been discussed, with a third of the diagnoses changed and treatment programs redesigned. There were forty-four surgical consultations, twenty-five on psychological matters, ten on infectious disease, thirty-three on diagnostic visualization, twenty-four on burns, sixteen on vascular medicine, five on endocrinology, six on ophthalmology, four on neurology, twenty-five on urology and six related to dialysis. NASA's domestic partners in the consultations included hundreds of doctors at the Uniformed Services University of Health Sciences in Bethesda, Maryland; the Maryland Institute for Emergency Medical Services Systems; The University of Texas Health Science Center in Houston, Texas; and LDS (formerly Latter Day Saints) Hospital in Salt Lake City, Utah. Soviet partners included more than sixty lecturers at the Yerevan Medical Institute of Advanced Physician Training and fifty directors of various medical institutions.

At first, many of them harbored a concern that having consulting specialists at multiple sites would lead to confusion or even the contradiction of one another's diagnoses. Instead, the opposite happened. Dr. Bruce Houtchens, a central figure in the Spacebridge consultations, recalls, "The American physicians, at least, said one of the things they missed when the Spacebridge program was terminated with Armenia—where we were, in fact, doing real patient consultations—was the lack of contact and critique by their peers in a real-time, on-line fashion."

They and their Soviet colleagues recommended to their respective governments that international agreements allowing for consultations after a disaster should always be in place. That suggestion still sits in political limbo, but the Spacebridge itself was reborn, anyway.

Heavy rainfall and heavy traffic on both ends of the link caused participants to be late for the final in a series of eighteen Telemedicine Spacebridges between the United States and Russia. American doctors at the Washington, DC site faced morning rush hour, while in Russia, eight hours ahead, flooding conditions trapped people in offices and on closed roads. It was June 24, 1994, and a historic phase in the evolution of international telemedicine was about to end.

The collection of medical specialists in Moscow virtually matched the group seated in the auditorium at the Uniformed Services University of the Health Sciences (USUHS) in Bethesda, Maryland. Radiology, cardiology, pathology, dermatology, internal medicine—a range of specialties played into the final conference. Faces familiar to each other and to students of telemedicine participated, among them Jay Sanders of the Medical College of Georgia (MCG), and Ron Poropatich, the pulmonary critical care specialist who was the lead United States Army clinician in the Somalia and Croatia telemedicine deployments. The telemedicine consultation began with reflections on the success of the 9-month program, called "Spacebridge to Moscow."

The offspring of the 1989 Spacebridge, this effort was launched after 4 years of talking. After two international telemedicine conferences in 1990 and 1991, NASA and the Moscow Ministry of the Interior took steps to forge the partnership that would allow for a steady exchange of Russian and American medical expertise. In December 1992, a United States delegation traveled to Moscow and created and signed an agreement with Russian officials that established the protocols for future collaboration. A reciprocal delegation from Moscow arrived in February 1993 to visit all participating sites and to meet their American counterparts. The sites included several players in the first Spacebridge after the earthquake: USUHS; the University of Texas Health Sciences Center; NASA Medical Operations Branch, Johnson Space Center; LDS Hospital; the University of Utah Health Science Center; and Fairfax Hospital in Falls Church, Virginia.

At the American ground station, NASA's Lewis Research Center in Cleveland, Ohio locked on to Loutch, a former Russian military satellite used for communications with the Mir space station. Lewis then coordinated continental communications through a United States domestic satellite. That included encrypting broadcasts on the American side to ensure patient confidentiality.

While putting the technical infrastructure in place in the United States, in July 1993, an American delegation installed telemedicine equipment in the Clinical Hospital of the Medical Department of the Ministry of Interior. The Clinical Hospital is a 400-bed facility providing health care services to police, firefighters and retirees and their families.

A scant two months after the installation, with little time for technical checkouts, consultations in living color with two-way audio and two-way video began. Participants on the American side took turns hosting the events at their respective sites. On the Russian side, participants from the Clinical Hospital and the Moscow Medical Academy convened in the Hospital's auditorium.

The series of consultations covered clinical territory new to specialists in both nations. Medical discoveries and observations made after the Chernobyl nuclear reactor accident occupied the first session on September 10, 1993. As part of the exchange, the Russian team presented patients that they thought had cancer from radiation exposure. Some American physicians disagreed, claiming there could be other causes for the disease. That day, thinking on both sides of the ocean about the ramifications of the Chernobyl disaster moved forward.

Soon after, the Russians interrupted the scheduled programming with an urgent request to help those wounded in the coup attempt against President Boris Yeltsin. Among those hurt was an American journalist, who described his hideout, the shots that ultimately claimed his arm, and the bloody death of a friend who had tried to rescue him.

In the course of the Spacebridge sessions, opinions and new findings were presented. Russian physicians were using electrically driven devices in orthopedic rehabilitation and additional uses for ultrasound in diagnosis, and hyperbaric chambers in treatment. Whereas there are little more than a handful of hyperbaric treatment facilities in the United States—and these are used to treat decompression sickness such as a scuba diver's case of "the bends"—there are hundreds in use for multiple applications in Russia. Russian physicians learned from American diagnostic techniques in infectious disease and emergency medicine, for example. Sessions on space medicine prepared both sets of physicians for handling the problems seen on shuttle missions and the space station Mir, soon to be occupied by American as well as Russian astronauts.

In the final conference in June, United States Army physicians at Walter Reed Army Medical Center graphically demonstrated the diagnostic challenge of sarcoidosis, a chronic disease that can terribly effect both the inside and the outside of the body. Sarcoidosis, which affects a number or organs, seems peculiar to people of African descent. With the percentage of African Americans in the U.S. Army at somewhere around 28 percent, Army specialists have been compelled to improve their diagnostic and treatment expertise of it and to package that knowledge for doctors and medics in the field.

One patient had collapsed during routine physical training for his military duties and was rushed to the emergency room. The only irregularity found had surfaced during a cardiology examination on an EKG. Specialists reviewing the graph in Moscow detected the same aberration. Based on that alone, however, no one could make an accurate diagnosis.

The radiologist next attempted to target the various possibilities evident from a chest X-ray. On an X-ray, sarcoidosis appears very much like tuberculosis, although the course of the disease is entirely different. The image could have also indicated other respiratory afflictions. Still, there was no way a definite diagnosis could be made.

An electronic stethoscope, allowing Russian participants to hear the beating heart of the patient thousands of miles way, confirmed a heart problem. The cause, however, was still unknown.

Papules of normal skin color that were clustered on the patient's eyelid and surrounding the eye could have had many causes, including leprosy, so no conclusion could be drawn from looking at the skin with the naked eye. To refine the diagnosis, therefore, the dermatologist demonstrated the use of a rhinoscope and dermatoscope. These two instruments each use a very small camera, like the one used in laparoscopic surgeries. This scope-camera set-up actually gives a remote specialist using the telemedicine system a clearer, more open view of a site than the doctor with the patient performing the exam. In other words, the Russians could view the inside of the patient's nose and the condition of his skin better than the American using the instrument. Finally, the pathologist presented microscopic findings that confirmed the diagnosis of sarcoidosis. Again, by attaching the microscope to the tiny camera, the details of cell structure were perfectly clear to the Russians.

American and Russian physicians concluded their sessions with a look at lessons learned. Technical pitfalls had strained their patience throughout the program, with audio as well as video capabilities always in the realm of uncertainty. For example, the session on hyperbaric oxygen treatment abruptly recessed when Loutch, which is an older satellite, was shut down for an hour because of a lunar eclipse. Russian technicians had feared there would not be enough sunlight to charge its batteries during the eclipse, and that they might lose it.

Early in the process, Russian physicians had expressed their hope that the Telemedicine Spacebridges would give them insight into reaching underserved populations in the rural areas outside of Moscow. Like some of the very rural or frontier areas of Australia, the United States and other countries, however, a weak telecommunications infrastructure threatens to keep many Russians distanced from health care. Fortunately, MedTel Cominform is addressing the problem head on. MedTel is the private company transmuted from the Soyuzmedinform Scientific Production Agency of the former Soviet Union's Ministry of Health. In the hope of creating a network of short "spacebridges" throughout Russia, the company is developing portable satellite transceivers. Medical expertise could then be beamed from point to point, where the transceivers rested.

5

Healing on Farms and Frontiers

It's my opinion that telemedicine is of tremendous value in several aspects of health care. One, in making it possible to reach out into the rural area and provide state of the art medicine by that means. It also has tremendous value in elevating the standards of continuing medical education.

Michael DeBakey, MD
Chancellor, Baylor College of Medicine

Medicine at a distance is one of the most basic definitions of telemedicine. The practice may rely on satellite or ordinary telephone lines; it may involve interactive television or facsimile. Whatever the level of technological sophistication, the goal is the same: improved access to medical expertise. Throughout the world, Ken Bird and Max House inspired doctors serving distant populations to use technology to bring the patient closer to the doctor and to bring health care professionals closer to each other.

For two days in October 1982, pediatricians in New Delhi, India, conducted a feasibility experiment for national application of telemedicine. Eighty percent of India's 700 million people lived in rural areas or remote terrain, so the project offered the promise of radically changing healthcare for the entire country. From 600 miles away, specialists were able to examine sick children using two-way audio and video.

While generally satisfied with the results, the doctors felt that the sound quality fell short. The doctors had no confidence that the auditory transmissions allowed for reliable diagnoses of respiratory problems and certain heart problems. That problem has critical implications for telemedicine, namely, even a good network may not be good enough for specialists, who listen for subtle shifts in pitch and look for faint changes in hue. It's reminiscent of the Mayo Clinic's reasoning in configuring an expensive state-of-the art system. The Indian investigators also concluded the network was too expensive to take nationwide, so the two-day experiment remained just that.

A few years later, Australia used telemedicine to conquer the vast distances that separated many towns from modern health care. Part of the challenge was that 30,000 health department employees in the giant state of Queensland, stretching 1,300 miles north-south and 700 miles east-west, were spread among 1,010 locations.

With government sponsorship, a satellite network called the North-West Telemedicine Project began serving five isolated Queensland towns with a population of 3,890 people, most of whom were Aborigines or Torres Strait Islanders. Only four of the towns actually had hospitals, with two of them staffed by nurses alone. In an emergency, the gravely ill were shuttled by the Royal Flying Doctor Service airplane, also used to transport health care practitioners to the towns. In the first year of the telemedicine network's operation, the number of evacuations handled by the Royal Flying Doctor Service dropped from 215 to 174.

Of course, as Dr. Max House often reminds colleagues when he talks about the “glamorous television projects” of telemedicine’s early days, the cost of satellite and interactive video transmission put a lot of good projects out of business. After a brief hiatus, Australia rejuvenated telemedicine efforts in 1991. This time the starting point was terrestrially-based systems involving mostly the transmission of X-rays (so-called “teleradiology”).

In the United States, Montana can seem a lot like Queensland. Montanans laugh when their health care access problem is viewed as one common to rural communities in the United States. Fewer than 1 million people live in the state that ranks fourth largest in terms of land mass. Also, the state has no medical school, typically the headquarters for telemedicine activities in an area.

Jim Reid had a few words to give in response to the American officials who proposed to create “The Information Superhighway” throughout the country: “The Information Supergravel Road is in Montana.” The first director of the Eastern Montana Telemedicine Network, Reid had the odds against him when he set out to launch his project. He had no major funding, and, worse yet, he was a physician’s assistant preaching to doctors.

After four years of research and cajoling, Reid established a six-month, six-site trial centered at Deaconness Medical Center, a private, non-profit 272-bed hospital. Deaconness is in Billings, the largest city in a 500-mile radius. Only about 100,000 people live there.

At the time the network was launched in October 1993, physicians were flown sixty-five times a month to towns in the Deaconness service area of 121,000 square miles in a $4 million airplane. These were towns in Montana like Culbertson, Glendive, Miles City and Sidney, none of which had a psychiatrist and most of which lacked other specialists as well. On average, only two beds a day were occupied in the outlying hospitals. Everyone else who needed steady attention had to go to Billings.

Reid knew that after the six-month trial funded by Deaconness, the project could be derailed by expenses. Among the causes were the 320-mile distance between Deaconness and its farthest link in Culbertson for which the telephone company charged an outrageous $8,000 a month to keep the network running. Comparatively, the cost of doing the same kind of wiring in rural Georgia was $1,200 a month. The network relied on dedicated T1 lines which are bundles of phone lines capable of a wider range of transmissions.

Reid had a plan to move the network toward self-sufficiency. By promoting it as a free convenience for both medical and non-medical applications in the remote communities, he baited people who might be willing to pay for the "free" gift later. Businesses, for example, could go to the hospital to use the system for video conferences.

The scheme included customized surveys about the telemedicine trial for health care providers, patients, instructors, students, administrators, business users and anyone else who might have derived benefit from the program. The data, he hoped, would demonstrate the cost-effectiveness of the system by documenting its value in areas not traditionally included as "health care costs." These include travel time saved and travel-related expenses, including mileage, meals, lodging and wages. The wages have been described by Jane Preston of the Texas Telemedicine Project as, "salary spilled on the highway." As a result of the survey, Reid wanted people who did not have to travel to Deaconness, or who effectively used the video conference system, to realize its full value.

Logs of network activity during the trial show a unique pattern of use in relation to other networks, but one that Reid predicted for eastern Montana. As expected, the overwhelming number of consults provided mental health and psychiatric services. There were ninety-five such sessions *versus* the thirty-five for all other specialties combined. Ninety medical education programs were broadcast, one hundred administrative conferences were held, and business used the system for video conferences forty times. While the system was fundamentally intended to deliver health care to the frontier, it also brought valuable and marketable videoconferencing capability to the remote sites, making the rural hospital an "on-ramp" instead of an "off-ramp" for the nation's developing information superhighway.

In addition to the populations of the United States and Australia, even the people in a relatively small country with a strong history in state-managed health care, can have a problem accessing medical expertise. This was the case in Norway. However, Norwegian doctors had an aggressive plan to solve it. Dr. Steinar Pedersen, the first Head of the Department of Telemedicine at the University Hospital of Tromsø, outlined the failed approach:

> Many different types of benefits have been tried to make specialists stay in remote areas. Measures as an extra week of vacation, extra salary and extended possibilities to travel for meeting colleagues at

home and abroad have all been without success. The specialists state that professional isolation is the main reason for not wanting to practice in remote areas.

Norway certainly wasn't alone. Rural or remote communities in many countries face an identical, spiraling problem: Specialists have little or no desire to isolate themselves from modern techniques and the latest research by locating in a rural community; they stay where the intellectual action is. Family practitioners that *do* serve outlying regions experience the isolation, and even if they are doing their best, they may be using outdated or discarded therapies.

Without medical specialties in a hospital, patients are routinely moved to a medical center or university hospital, usually in a city. The result is a declining bed census in local hospitals. Communities atrophy when they face this year after year. As many towns in the rural United States have experienced, the hospital eventually shuts down. Losing a hospital means lost jobs, travel to visit sick loved ones and a blow to the spirit of the whole town.

Norway turned to technology for a solution. When government committed to use telemedicine to keep services alive for people in remote areas in February 1993, the Norwegian Minister of Health opened the Department of Telemedicine at the University Hospital of Tromsø. The hospital led an official charge to nurture medical competence in the field of telemedicine, and applications developed there will be spread throughout Norway's health care system. As part of its significant entry into the world of telemedicine, one of the Hospital's first activities was a May 1993 conference attended by 200 leaders of telemedicine programs from around the world.

Knowing something about the hierarchical structure of Norway's health care system helps in understanding how the country managed widespread implementation. An explanation appeared in *Telektronikk*, the technical journal of Norwegian Telecommunications, under whose direction the telemedicine system in northern Norway falls:

> The Norwegian public health services are decentralized and based on the principle of treatment on the lowest efficient level of care. The primary health service is the responsibility of the municipalities while the counties are responsible for the hospitals. Each county has a central hospital and a varying number of local hospitals. The country is divided into five health regions. Each region has a regional hospital with the responsibility of taking care of special medical competence and treatment. On a national level there are also some hospitals to take care of particularly rare or complicated types of illnesses.
>
> B. J. Nymo, *Telektronikk*, January 1, 1993

The geographic heart of the program is in the northern and sparsely populated area of the country. Services radiate from the University Hospital hundreds of miles north of the Arctic Circle to the primary care facilities serving 600,000 people spread over Norway's northern half, a long stretch of land on the Norwegian Sea. Eighty-six percent of the country's 4.3 million people reside in the southern region closer to Oslo. The distance between Tromsø and Oslo equals the distance between Oslo and Rome, Italy. In the more populous areas, physician-to-population ratios are similar to those in the United States, with one specialist and one general practitioner for every 291 people. In the northern area now served by telemedicine, however, the ratio is 1 to 1194.

The current focus of consultations between remote physicians and Tromsø specialists is in the areas of otorhinolaryngology, dermatology and psychiatry. Medical outreach has been extended on an occasional basis to a bordering town in Russia.

Outside of the context of the developing national telemedicine network, a demonstration project was established jointly by American, British and Norwegian business interests at the 1994 Winter Olympics in Lillehammer, near Oslo. The experiment electronically linked specialists to Hamar and Gjovik, where the skating events were held. Fortunately, even though the resource was never needed, the availability drew some international attention to the value of telemedicine.

It some ways, it would appear that the Norwegian program does not have the financial pitfalls of telemedicine in the United States, but it isn't true across the board. At least for the present, Norwegian specialists have a reimbursement issue with the government.

As part of a plan to give doctors an incentive to bring health care to remote citizens, Norway has been providing special compensation for the physicians who travel to them. While specialists utilizing the telemedicine network to serve those populations may actually help a greater number of patients, the fact that they are not traveling actually reduces their income.

The impact of the European Economic Agreement, which created the European Economic Community, had not yet been felt in a significant way in the Norwegian program. The expectation, however, is that it will nurture joint projects in medical research and development long before it leads to ongoing teleconsultation relationships across national borders.

In the meantime, the Space Age has given rise to steady international cooperation in advancing telemedicine.

6

Space Clinics

Telemedicine is not only important for terrestrial care, but for extraterrestrial practice in the future of space medicine. I believe in order for earthlings to survive, we're going to have to have a system of evaluating illnesses in space and being able to corroborate that through telemedicine.

Astronaut Bernard A. Harris, Jr., MD

Bernard Harris's doctor bag was a clear plastic pouch sealed with Velcro. He removed a stethoscope and began the examination. Charlie Precourt, his patient, bobbed away from the doctor with each touch. He would have floated completely out of range if untethered. As Dr. Harris proceeded, a gold medallion escaped from his shirt and seemed to swim in front of his face. The patient looked relaxed, with a little sway in his back and arms dangling at his side. In fact, Precourt's posture was reminiscent of pictures of prehistoric man. Dr. Harris checked one thing after another. He found fluid on the lungs, the heart migrating toward the center of the chest and other organs shifting and hiding. In short, Charlie was perfectly normal—under the circumstances.

Charlie Precourt's checkup in microgravity occurred twenty years after the first medical doctor experienced space travel. It was historic as an in-orbit physical examination. Broadcasting it from a space shuttle to the Mayo Clinic was an equally historic telemedicine experiment.

The events occurred aboard the space shuttle Columbia during her April 26 to May 6, 1993 flight, jointly sponsored by Germany and the United States. It was on May 4, 1993 when Harris and an earthbound group of colleagues conferred about the physiological effects of microgravity.

One of a dozen active astronaut-physicians in the American shuttle program, Dr. Harris hung his shingle near a single rack on the side of the spacecraft that held enough equipment to supply an emergency room—a mass spectrometer for pulmonary function tests, echocardiogram for images of the heart, electrocardiogram for reviewing heart waves and an ergometer for exercise stress tests. Part of the daily routine involved drawing over a liter of blood, which was spun down on a centrifuge and put in the freezer for transport back to Earth.

Astronauts always come home showing the side effects of microgravity, but there is some uncertainty about what is normal and what is actually a space illness. Fifty to sixty percent of astronauts would have no uncertainty about how to classify their neurovestibular destabilization—motion sickness. "Normal" adjustments to the zero-gravity condition include fluid shifts to the head. Astronauts can feel the onset of that edema, which causes obvious facial puffiness. In the first couple days, they lose a liter or two of body fluid, the heart shrinks, muscle atrophies and bone disappears. Some studies show this happens at the rate of 1 percent a month. While the scientific term for the collection of effects is Space Adaptation Syndrome (SAS), a more popular phrase is "fat face and chicken legs." It describes exactly what they see in each other: The dramatic upward movement of fluid in microgravity makes the legs look skinny and the face look fat.

In the telemedicine conference, Dr. Harris pointed out that the physical examination was the physician's first tool, but it took decades to give it a role in studying human physiology in orbit. The study conducted in the United States-Germany mission was designed to use the physical exam to collect better data on SAS. The three objectives were to methodically evaluate every system of the body, to direct research toward the areas of significant change and finally, in the process of discovering what happens to the human body and documenting it through a physical examination, to standardize physical exams for the future practice of space medicine.

During the link, Dr. Harris emphasized that a study like this gives physicians "an idea of what normal is all about, what normal space physiology is, and what it will be like in the future." One added benefit is preparation for the medical problems that will affect travelers to the moon and future travelers to Mars, among other places.

The relevance of this study and other in-orbit biological research spans multiple medical disciplines. For example, decreased bone mass leads to osteoporosis—an affliction of many older people, as well as others with particular degenerative diseases. All astronauts returning to normal gravity experience such extreme lightheadedness that they need help to stand. Also, lymphocytes stop duplicating, especially the important lymphocyte in fighting AIDS and HIV. No one really knows what prolonged space flight will do to the depletion or production of them. Will it raise the astronauts' susceptibility to disease?

At this stage of discovery, only the most basic physiological cause and effect relationships have been established and outlined by NASA, as follows:

Causes	*Effects*
fluid shifts bone demineralization muscle loss electrolyte changes cardiac deconditioning	kidney stones fractures cardiac arrhythmias constipation
closed-loop confined environment	eye problems infectious disease skin problems toxic exposures
construction in space and space walks	trauma decompression sickness
accidents	burns toxic exposures radiation
other	space motion sickness

Results of the non-human telemedical science experiments also conducted aboard the shuttles will undoubtedly help answer some of the other questions about the effects of space on human physiology.

This is mission control. The Endevour is now crossing the Atlantic Ocean. These are live television downlinks of the Space Tissue Loss experiment. These are views of some of the cell growth cultures under microscope.

Johnson Space Center, Texas, April 1994

Astronaut Michael R.U. Clifford maneuvered a tiny camera from chamber to chamber showing live microscopic tissue samples of fish embryos, while the footage was being viewed by scientist on earth. In one view, the tiny heart beat regularly. The eyes of the fish seemed to be of normal size and placement. The curvature of the tail and embryonic red blood cells coursing through a flimsy body in its first days of life were evident. The next embryo, also four days old, had an elongated and flattened heart with an irregular beat; it had no eyes. In fact, two of the three live embryos on board developed abnormalities.

Col. Bill Wiessman, MD scrutinized the footage. It was his team at the Walter Reed Institute of Research that designed the fish egg experiment with NASA scientists. Did the lack of gravity affect how the heart developed? he wondered. What does that mean for men and women in space?

Wiessman played the tape over and over. Astronaut Clifford announced the historic broadcast with customary restraint:

You've got the blue shift of Endeavour on call here. While the blue shift's been performing their jobs up here on flight deck, we've had a couple other experiments working on mid-deck called Space Tissue Loss. Most of these experiments involve growing live cells in a microgravity environment . . . experiments show some interesting effects of how microgravity does slow down the rate of muscle and bone regeneration . . . (It) is the first flight of the video microscope, which allows the investigator on the ground to interact with this equipment and the crew members up here. We're looking for some interesting results.

The live television downlink of the Space Tissue Loss experiment is one of a series of projects that might be called "telemedical science" in space. In this case, researchers on the ground used images and data beamed from Endeavour to further investigate the effects of microgravity on muscle and bone cells. By understanding what happens on the cellular level in the on-board fish embryos, they hoped to advance understanding of what happens to humans on the cellular level.

Their hypothesis is that discoveries in space, such as those made on and by Bernard Harris on Columbia, will help the earthbound as well as astronauts: While astronauts suffer from bone loss and muscle deterioration, or deconditioning, in space flight, the same effect shows up in some recuperating trauma patients whose ability to regenerate bone and muscle is somehow impaired. If a therapy that cures the microgravity effect could be found, perhaps it would translate into a cure for the trauma patient.

On its maiden voyage, the video microscope fit comfortably with the other experiments, tools and lockers that stacked seven high on the mid-deck. More precisely, the camera was called a direct digital and analog imager. The instrument had to fit weight and height specifications for on-board units. At 19 inches long by 17 inches wide by 9.5 inches high and weighing a few pounds less than the 70-pound limit, the successful use of the device signaled numerous possibilities for telemedicine in space. The video microscope points to a capability for doing infectious disease and opthalmologic consultations from space. The same thing can be done over vast distances on Earth, where NASA practiced.

NASA's interest in telemedicine, and that of space ministries everywhere, dates back to the first manned launches. This is because the agency is in the unique position of providing health care to the most remote people—those in space. The design of telemedicine programs involving space travel have always reflected a dual application to earth and space medicine. Going back to NASA's projects with Native Americans in the 1970s, the instruments and transmission modalities used and the lessons learned have held value for the earthbound as well as the orbiting.

About the same time that Ken Bird's pioneering work got underway at Massachusetts General Hospital, NASA entered the telemedicine scene. Paradoxically, the motives for both efforts were different, yet identical. They were different in the sense that Bird integrated technology that was readily available, whereas NASA launched projects to serve as tests for new space technology. They were identical in the sense that both aimed to use technology to bring the best medicine available to distant and underserved populations.

In 1973, NASA launched the most enduring of its trials to electronically bring health care to the Papago Indian Reservation in the Sonora Desert south of Tucson, Arizona. Called Space Technology Applied to Rural Papago Advanced Health Care (STARPAHC), the project married the expertise of Lockheed Corporation, Indian Health Service and the space agency. As with the other NASA projects, the goal was to test systems that could send data back about astronauts engaged in long duration space missions.

Underlying the goal was a premise that many similarities exist between administering quality health care in space and to remote populations on Earth. Among the similarities are limited access to medical expertise and clinical equipment and lack of adequate surgical and therapeutic facilities. Further, transmitting an X-ray via microwave from a spacecraft to a ground station is very much like transmitting from one ground station to another. STARPAHC, therefore, used two-way microwave television to connect a van on the reservation to two hospitals—basically the same arrangement used in Massachusetts.

Staffed by Indian paramedics, the mobile exam room was equipped with an X-ray machine, electrocardiograph and advanced bioinstrumentation intended for monitoring the status of astronauts. Under the supervision of doctors based in Sells, Arizona, the paramedics administered health care to more than 10,000 people on and near the 4,300-square-mile reservation. Site selection for the project hinged in large part on the Papago community's willingness to accept primary care from physician's assistants—an accepted practice in Arizona—and a commitment to support the system after the test period was completed, which they managed to do for nearly 15 years after NASA stopped supporting the program in 1978.

STARPAHC represents a pace-setting telemedicine project benefiting from a partnership of public and private sector expertise. It was organized following a scientific approach to the challenge of remote health care delivery. And, at the outset, it had in place an evaluative process, allowing STARPAHC participants to feed medical data and systems performance information into a database of the Indian Health Service. Finally, it is truly distinguished because it involved the Papago people themselves in the system design and development of a criteria for performance.

Another demonstration project temporarily served Native Alaskans in fourteen villages with daily telemedicine consultations from a hospital in Tanana. The communications system was also used for communications between patients hospitalized in Tanana and their families back in the villages.

STARPAHC and the Spacebridge to Moscow helped prepare the international community for the routine practice of medicine in space. Certainly, the Spacebridge provided unique insights into space medicine since Russian specialists could share nearly seven years of human habitation of the space station Mir. Also, during its series of solo efforts and collaborative missions with other nations, NASA built up on-board readiness to handle sickness and injury.

When the space program began in the 1960s, the astronauts traveled light, medically speaking. In the Mercury Program, although the risk of medical problems was very high, the medical kit was small and basic—it contained only four medications. The Gemini package was called the In-flight Medical Accessory Kit, a collection of pre-packaged pharmaceuticals, topicals, injectibles, eyedrops and antibiotics. The drugs were mostly aimed at easing the effects of motion sickness and suppressing pain. The longer mission duration of Apollo flights, including one to the moon, necessitated expanded in-flight medical capability. During the 7,500 hours of flight time associated with the program space motion sickness and cardiac arrythmias had been amply documented.

A crippled Apollo 13 also drew attention to the impact of system failures on crew health and the need to consider life-support degradation or failure in the design of in-flight medical care systems. With Skylab, a rack of medical and dental hardware called the In-flight Medical Support System was added. Shuttle missions carry a Shuttle Orbiter Medical System which contains both diagnostic and therapeutic items including medications, bandages, an emergency medicine kit, a resuscitator and a contaminant cleanup kit.

The configuration of in-flight medical care and the use of telemedicine in space are determined by how long the mission is; the relative danger of mission objectives, such as a lot of extra-vehicular activity; a lot of laboratory science; construction activities on the lunar surface; and so on. As a corollary, the farther astronauts are from getting home quickly, the more autonomous their medical care needs to be. One exception, however, is the shuttle (high orbit) as compared to the space station (low orbit). The shuttle orbits the earth once every ninety minutes and has the capability to return to an appropriate landing area on Earth in a half of a day to a day, whereas personnel on board the space station might have a delay of a day or two.

Thus, telemedicine is much more likely to be an integral part of medical support on a space station than on Mars, which is about a year away in travel time. This may sound backwards at first, considering that telemedicine is all about reaching underserved and remote populations. Who could be more remote than astronauts on Mars? But, just as transmission dilemmas inhibit the functionality of many systems on Earth, the problem of communicating with Mars to conduct telemedicine is daunting. In short, it could never be used in an emergency situation. Here is what would happen:

Astronaut 1: "Mission control, John had an accident and is bleeding profusely from the upper leg. Please advise."

Eighteen minutes later Mission Control gets the message. Eighteen minutes after that, Astronaut 1 hears:

Mission Control: "Sounds like he hit the femoral artery. He's gonna need a lot of blood or he'll die."

Again, roughly 36 minutes later, the Mars transmission is received:

Astronaut 1: "Thanks mission control. That's become obvious to us."

So instead of relying on telemedicine for diagnosis and treatment guidance in anything less than an hour, NASA has conceptually put together a highly autonomous medical system to support Mars pioneers for about a year. This would include the capability to do major surgeries.

In 1984, during the Reagan Administration, when America's political power proposed Space Station Freedom, NASA went to work designing a station medical facility. In the original plan, Freedom was scheduled for construction in late 1994 or early 1995.

Based on the previous experiences with orbiting spacecraft, NASA decided to develop a suite of medical hardware called the Health Maintenance Facility (HMF). The plan was to include exercise equipment, dental and surgical supplies, anesthesia, pharmaceutical supplies to allow residents to make their own intravenous solutions, vital monitoring instruments and a Sterile Water Injection System (SWIS) which takes drinking water into one end and spits out sterile water at the other. The exercise countermeasure facility was to have a treadmill, bicycle ergometer and rowing machine with instrumentation to give the space station dweller the sense of rowing competitively. The vision included a computer which could be connected to on-board instruments and record and update patient records.

Just before it would have gone into a construction phase, Space Station Freedom was shelved because of shifting United States political priorities, and a phased approach was taken to development of the HMF. In lieu of creating a station bearing only the stars and stripes, the United States elected to team up with Russia and utilize the Mir, completed in March 1986 and occupied since February 1987. As many as ten shuttles to the Mir are planned to begin in May 1995, with American astronauts expected to stay up to ninety days. Collaboration among ESA, the Russian Space Agency (RSK), the United States, Japan and Canada will produce the International Space Station Alpha (ISSA) in 1997. It is expected to reside about two-hundred nautical miles away, in low earth orbit, at fifty-six degrees off the equator—a configuration very similar to Mir's. NASA went back to the drawing board to revise designs for a new space station medical facility and to determine what enhancements to Mir's medical capability might be desirable.

Ambitious EUROMIR missions, putting European Space Agency (ESA) astronauts on board the Mir, began in 1994. This was well in advance of the American ones. When German Ulf Merhold, who was the first non-American to fly aboard a U.S. space shuttle, set his sights on the Mir, his daily work schedule for a month included six hours of experiments. At fifty-three, Merhold was one of the most experienced space travelers when he went to Mir armed with the largest quantity of biological samples ever taken into space—thirty-five pounds of frozen blood, urine and saliva. Almost all of his research focused on human physiology. The mission was one of two that cost ESA almost $53 million.

A scaled-down version of the Crew Health Care System (CHCS, pronounced "checks") has evolved as the model for the first space station medical facility. Changes to it have kept pace with the seven revisions of the space station's design as a whole. One of the things that could not be deleted was a Crew Medical Restraint System, a kind of blanket with belts that holds the patient in one spot and contains required equipment. Tabs on the restraint system fit into tracks on the floor, wall lockers or other non-moving components of the spacecraft, holding the system in place. This is an important requirement in a microgravity environment, where the physician's touch actually pushes an unrestrained patient away. In space, even if the crew medic sits on someone's chest to do compression, every time there is a push, the patient moves. Without restraint, there is no way to create the force necessary to perform life-saving resuscitation maneuvers.

A second important part of CHCS is the Environmental Health System, a monitoring system which includes a microbial air sampler and combustion product analyzer. Using the air sampler, an astronaut can collect organisms in the air and grow them in a special on-board incubator for further observation. The combustion product analyzer is an upscale cousin of the household smoke detector with monitors that provide a warning about hazardous levels of chemicals. On a space station, it could be connected to a caution and warning system, so if it did detect a fire or situation that could lead to a fire, personnel on board would have ample notice.

A practical example of using this kind of portable warning system in preserving crew health is after extra-vehicular activity—that is, a stroll in open space. Hydrazine is the propellant used in the orbit maneuvering system engines, the small rockets used to thrust the spacecraft into a slightly different position and perhaps to get closer to a satellite that the crew will repair. If inhaled, hydrazine kills; even a small amount will do great harm to a human being. As a precautionary measure to burn off any crystallized hydrazine on a space suit used in open space, the astronaut will face the sun. When the astronaut returns to the airlock and pressure starts to return to normal, any remaining crystals sublimate and fill the room with vapor. The CHCS monitor can then tell instantly if the dangerous chemical is present.

While the clinical hardware for the space station's medical care facility sounds as if it is "designed to specifications"—the government's way of saying that it's expensive—the total cost in phase one is $60 million. For the most part, it is standard government-furnished equipment, that is, commercial off-the-shelf units modified for space flight. This is a very different scenario from that of the early 1960s, when had to invent technological solutions that did not yet exist.

With the space station in a low earth orbit, the perceptible delay in communications between the high-orbit shuttle and Earth would not be present. If Dr. Bernard Harris were to utter, "Here is Charlie's heart," from a low earth orbit, it could sound as if he were in the same room. The broadcast from the shuttle, however, had a second or so delay. Real-time telemedicine, including real-time remote surgery, is therefore in the realm of possibility for the space station.

Surgery in space is never easy, though.

A surgical suite on board the space station would have features unheard of in terrestrial medicine. Over the years, experiments in simulated microgravity have shown what techniques are needed to cope with the unusual process of surgery in space. Under normal circumstances, blood will spurt out of a severed artery. If a vein is cut, the blood dribbles out. In space, it doesn't matter if the severed vessel is an artery or a vein; the blood heads out and upward. Specifically, if an artery is hit, the blood becomes a projectile. Blood pouring out of the vein forms globules that rise gently toward the ceiling. Without a containment mechanism for the flying and floating fluids, tissue and other body fragments, a surgeon would have to fend them off during the procedure.

A laminar flow device, situated over the patient, solves the problem in all situations except the nicked artery. It creates a constant jet of air over the body, blowing one way and drawing particles into itself. Any airborne matter, whether shavings from a dental procedure or venous blood, would be caught in the airstream and removed from the environment.

On the space station, there will eventually be a comprehensive telemedicine capability to reinforce in-flight care. Real-time, two-way audio and video and a range of attached examination instruments will be used routinely. Even in preparation for the American occupation of Mir, telemedicine is playing an important role. A communication link joins the Russian training facility in Star City outside of Moscow and in Texas. That ground link hints at the kind of contact American space station inhabitants will probably maintain with Russian and American colleagues after they get on board.

Since options for the ride home from Mir are limited, certain other health care considerations come into play. Crew rely on transport modules that detach from the space station and fall to earth the way early Apollo capsules did. There is some danger with this, as well as with shuttle landings after prolonged flight because of the deconditioning effects of microgravity on the human body. Even when exercise countermeasures to ward off the effects of space flight are used, extended time in space leaves an astronaut weak, if not incapacitated, in the legs. The most extreme example is cosmonaut Musa H. Manarov, who lived in Mir for 366 days. Right after he landed and asked for a cigarette, he had to be carried out of the module. In the event of an emergency, such as a crash landing, astronauts would have be able to get up and get out on their own power.

The current program of experiments during shuttle missions of ever-increasing duration will help physicians anticipate the range of astronauts' physiological problems. the experiments will help doctors design countermeasures, and, as an integral element of the health care delivery system in space, establish an ongoing role for telemedicine on the space station as well as on future shuttle missions.

Dr. Harris likes to point out that the roots of telemedicine are really in space. Without the strides in telecommunications spawned by the space program and defense industry in various countries, telemedicine wouldn't exist. Space and defense research have led and continue to lead the technological advances that will transform the quality of health care for remote populations on Earth and travelers in space.

7

Digital Age Wonders

Medical technology will keep leaping forward because it is good for the patients, and because the technology is available.

Danny Cohen
computer scientist
The Rand Corporation

One in three—those are the odds of contracting some form of cancer. One in four people, in most modern countries, will die of it. Trained on this family of killers is an army of weapons of the Space Age, Information Age and Digital Age—three ways of characterizing the final decades of the twentieth century.

Cancer comes in so many forms that the devices and techniques used to fight it give a good sense of the range of current medical innovations. They also walk us into the future of health care, when many presently discouraging statistics will change.

One tale from health care's past has become an all-too-familiar nightmare: Emma's X-ray showed a cluster of dots, too faint to be felt yet by the radiologist. Eight months later, terror gripped the patient—she had a deadly tumor in her left breast. After surgery stripped her of her breast, chemotherapy took away her hair. She died within the year.

The technology that is helping to change this sad story has ties to military readiness (early detection), space travel (diagnosis) and nature (cure and prevention). The same kind of technology that advances the war on breast cancer has even broader applications in conquering other forms of cancer and non-cancer diseases.

When the young women of today go to the doctor for their first mammogram, the specialists will look at a computer screen, not a film, to make a diagnosis. That doctor could be in the next room or in another country, since the image will be transmitted electronically. Regardless of location, the clarity of the image will be better than that of a film X-ray.

Actually, using the future tense in this scenario is not necessary. The shift toward direct digital imaging has begun to take hold around the world, both in academic and in military medicine. Filmless radiology, giving rise to teleradiology networks, is where X-ray technology is headed. Imaging subspecialties such as telemammography are included in this move away from messy developing chemicals and the quality and filing problems of film.

Georgetown University in Washington, DC is a leader in pointing the way toward use of digital mammography, including its use in telemedicine. What Matthew Freedman, MD and Seong K. Mun, PhD are developing there flows from a decade of work done by Japanese researchers at the Fuji Corporation, which combined its equipment innovations with patented technology licensed from the Eastman Kodak Company in the early 1980s.

There are a number of expected advantages of digital mammography. The biggest is that there is hope that the image of a woman's breast will finally give a clear picture of either health or malignancy. In digital mammography, the computer is used to enhance the image in order to make it much easier for a radiologist to detect tiny spots in the picture. This is also referred to as image processing, different than a description given in Chapter 9 of a direct digital imager's dynamic range adjustment, which refers to exposure correction. By changing the appearance of the image, image processing allows indications of the disease to actually become more obvious.

Another element that has worked well in the lab is the computer's capacity to look at an image and analyze it. The computer is programmed to look for predetermined signs that may then help the radiologist find cancer. The third advantage of image processing is that, since the image is in digital form, it can be transmitted—without degradation of resolution—to another location for diagnostic consultation or medical education purposes.

There are different ways of creating a digital mammogram. One utilizes a refrigerator-sized unit that performs direct digital mammography. What the patient sees is something like the X-ray machine in standard mammography, with a cassette that holds a digital receptor. The cassette is later fed to a special digital plate reader that gets the information off the plate and puts it in digital form. At that point, it can be sent to the computer. Unfortunately, the imager's large size also hints at the price, which hovers around $200,000.

The second method of creating a digital mammogram is scanning the standard mammogram film to put it into digital form. Roughly the size of a large desktop computer, this

$50,000 scanner far exceeds the performance characteristics of normal office models, which, at the high end, cost about $15,000. Most certainly, however, the tools of digital mammography will follow the same path as other medical technology, in that advances in miniaturization, driven by user demand for portability, will lead to a reduction in size and cost.

The impetus and funding for the Georgetown effort comes from the United States military. Telemedical applications relate to the fact that the military organizations have women stationed at bases all over the world, but only a few of those bases have radiologists who specialize in mammography.

Similarly, in the rural and remote areas of many countries there are health care practitioners who are capable of capturing the image but not necessarily interpreting it. Once the mammogram is captured in digital form, the computer can be used to search the picture for abnormalities and to point them out to the physician. This process is called computer-aided diagnosis, and it is a fundamental kind of progress in the realm of telemedicine.

Digital mammography also offers the hope to women under 50 years of age that the image will be clear enough to make early detection realistic. The problem with film X-rays of younger women is that their breast tissue's density affects image clarity, so catching a pre-cancerous indication or an early cancer in them is very difficult.

In trying to prove that the quality of digital mammography is better than conventional film images, studies have focused on the detection of calcifications. A mammogram often depicts dense, white dots, which are the images of calcifications. Normally, these are dispersed and few. Radiologists now know that a cluster of them is suspicious and can indicate a malignancy.

On a standard image, this kind of cluster of eight or ten micro-calcifications may appear as indiscernible dots in a gray mass. An image in digital format, however, can reveal pinpoints of light easily seen through contrast enhancement, spatial frequency filtering and magnification.

After the woman's mammogram reveals a suspicious shape or she feels a lump herself, she has to find out quickly if there is a malignancy. Among the picture-taking devices present on the Hubble Telescope, there is one based on technology that can also change the way a biopsy is done. For this procedure, the patient goes into a room adjoining her doctor's office and lies prostrate on a table that allows the breast to poke through a hole. The doctor takes a needle, goes into the breast where there is a tumor suspected and illuminates it without involving the entire breast. All the work is done below the plane of the body, where the breast protrudes through the table. There is no invasion, no delay.

In the cancer fight, technology has also helped nature yield curative secrets, and the human body to yield clues to prevention. Taxol, found mainly in the bark of the Pacific yew tree, has been targeted as a possible cure, or at least an effective treatment for breast cancer, ovarian cancer, glioblastoma—the deadliest form of brain cancer—and malaria. Taxol fights tumor growth by disrupting the mitosis, or cell division, of the cancer. Clinical trials trying to prove its efficacy started springing up in 1994. Unfortunately, the destruction of mature trees to obtain the necessary material runs counter to sound environmental practices. As a result, researchers have had to select yew cells from various plants and cultivate them in a bioreactor.

Taxol, found naturally, offers only weak hope for cancer victims because of its limited availability and strength.

However, as cultivated by technological innovators, mostly in Korea and the United States, taxol's concentration is at least two orders of magnitude higher and environmentally acceptable.

The pervasive desire in research, and in all medicine, is prevention. Gene mapping, a process of locating and cataloguing genes, is integral to the prevention effort. Theoretically, once a gene's role in human physiology is known, it can be manipulated, or engineered, to alter the course of a person's health.

In 1994, Human Genome Sciences discovered that several genes it catalogued were linked with colon cancer. Earlier discoveries had targeted diseases known to be genetic, such as muscular dystrophy and cystic fibrosis. The powerful technology that helps researchers analyze data, create three-dimensional simulations and transmit data to colleagues is fundamental to the success of the search. Nevertheless, the process is tedious and costly. Identifying the gene that causes cystic fibrosis was a $150 million proposition.

Human genes are not the only ones that offer answers to human problems. The genetic map of the roundworm aided in the 1992 discovery that a particular cancer-causing gene affects the division and function of cells during normal development.

Eventually, so-called bioscience technology, such as genetic engineering and cell therapy, will supplant conventional drugs. It is part of a critical shift in health care from treating symptoms to arresting the underlying cause of disease.

In an area adjoining the operating room, Gail Evans, a patient, waits for surgery. A nurse is taking pictures of the gastrointestinal tract. She inserts a tiny robot into the patient's rectum. On the television screen in the operating room, where surgeons wait, the pictures appear.

In flexible endoscopy, involving the insertion of a scope into the digestive tract, the only active portion of the instrument is the tip. The scope includes an insertion tube, which is used to push the tip through the winding intestinal passageways. In the near future, a micro-robot will substituted for the working tip. Inserted into the rectum, it will be electronically controlled with a lever, or joystick, from a workstation.

By 1991, such "robot insects" were emerging as promising diagnostic and surgical tools. Since they are a digital device—meaning the images they capture can go straight into a computer or over a network to another location—they have myriad implications for telemedicine.

Small robots, or robotized instruments, are performing delicate biopsies in Switzerland. At the Swiss Federal Institute of Technology's Institute of Microengineering, researchers have also developed robot probes for implantation of capsules containing live cells. These cells produce the active substance which is directly administered at the site to be treated. The procedure requires extraordinary accuracy, but another achievement of the robots is their predictable handling of very fragile materials.

There are now machines small enough to swallow that can comfortably explore, photograph and transmit photos of the twists and tight spaces in a human body, such as the gastrointestinal tract. They could function as peripherals of a telemedicine system, just as small cameras now enable the otoscope, microscope, endoscope and others to interface with an interactive television set-up. Equipped with sensors to detect changes in pressure, temperature density and so on, the functionality of these robot insects goes far beyond that of an endoscope. From "Genghis Khan" to "Atilla" to "Squirt" to "Goliath"—the names of first, second, third and fourth generation miniature robots produced at the Massachusetts Institute of Technology in Boston—they're getting smarter and smaller. The smallest at this stage of development can be cupped in the palm of a hand.

At the other end of the spectrum is "Robodoc," a comparatively large addition to the hospital staff. Robodoc's particular specialty is hip replacements, but watching this expert at work gives a strong sense of how precisely Robodoc's "colleagues" could excise tumors, for example.

Robodoc tackled its first surgery on November 7, 1992. As the operating room team prepared, a computer monitor warned them: "DO NOT TOUCH ROBOT OR FIXTURES. PERFORMING BONE MOTION MONITOR TEST. PLEASE WAIT." Robodoc flexed its drilling arm, then stood still while two masked assistants dressed it in a clear plastic, flexible suit. The monitor flashed instructions: "GUIDE PROBE TO INSTALLATION VERIFICATION POINT ON FIXATOR EXTENSION ARM."

Meanwhile, in preparing the patient, Seth Cordova, for the historic operation, orthopedic surgeon William Bargar slit the man's flesh above the hip bone. Bargar then retracted the bloody mass of skin and muscle, exposing the underlying bone. The monitor issued new instructions: "MOVE ROBOT INTO POSITION BY OPERATING TABLE AND LOCK THE BASE." Two people rolled the 300-pound robot into position. The monitor next read: "REMOVE PIN EXTENDER AND GUIDE PROBE TO CENTER OF PIN HEAD." Bargar's gloved hands, splattered with blood, slipped the probe into a thin shaft. Robodoc's arm rotated and squarely approached its target. The operating room filled with the sound of drilling—that grating noise of invasion that seems like it should be far from a human being. With the monitor graphically indicating current depth, the team stood by while the drilling and irrigation continued. Finally, it read, “ROBOT PROCEDURE COMPLETE.”

Robodoc had succeeded in making a cementless implantation a more predictable event by coring the patient’s femoral shaft to accept a prosthesis precisely. It was the first active robotic device to perform an invasive surgical procedure based directly upon input from a computerized preoperative planning system. That system involved using CAT scans to map the femur precisely to the implant. This data in the computer was then fed to the robot, which was armed with an orthopedic drill.

The creation of Bargar and veterinarian Howard Paul, Robodoc is really only 35 inches tall, but is mounted on a 3.5-foot high base to bring its height above the patient and its weight to 300 pounds. This is a necessity if the robotic arm is to have the leverage to bore a clean cavity. The $575,000 “surgical assistant” began life in 1986 as part of a collaborative research project between IBM’s Thomas J. Watson Research Center, IBM’s Scientific Center and the University of California at Davis. Bargar and Paul’s company, Integrated Surgical Systems Inc. of Sacramento, California, has three Robodocs scheduled for 300 hip replacements in 1994 and 1995 as part of an extensive American test program to secure final approval for widespread use. This kind of system is used routinely in veterinary procedures in Sacramento, California as part of an extensive United States Food and Drug Administration (FDA) test program to secure final approval for widespread use. This kind of system is used routinely in veterinary procedures in Sacramento, California.

In a surgical context, robots are categorized very much like people: intelligent or non-intelligent; independent or completely dependent. A tele-operation system is a precisely matched, 1 to 1 replication of a leader and follower analogy. When the surgeon controlling the leader moves, the remote follower moves precisely in consonance. To pick up a scalpel, the surgeon grabs the leader, performs the movement of picking up a scalpel, and the non-intelligent follower picks it up in exactly the same way. This ostensibly simple arrangement is central to the telepresence, or remote, surgical system.

Building on the tele-operation model is also a technique known as "telerobotics," which gives the follower its own intelligence. This is the model for Robodoc. If the same motion of picking up a scalpel is performed in a telerobotic environment, the surgeon types or speaks instructions that send a signal to the robot's hand. In a sense, the robot says to itself: "Ah-ha! Pick up!" and it grasps the scalpel. Often equipped with image recognition systems, the robots—or intelligent followers—can find objects, recognize them, pick them up and perform certain functions to and with them.

If the clinical telerobotic systems of today rely on intelligent robots, those of tomorrow's telemedicine will be "geniuses." Mid-1990's robots can only bring the kind of replicable precision to surgical tasks that human beings themselves cannot guarantee. The affordability of telerobotic surgery centers on the fact that more accuracy and speed means less problems and expense such as blood loss, operating room time and the risk of having to repeat a procedure. In the area of hip replacements, for example, roughly 35,000 revisions are done each year in the United States alone. One could buy millions of intelligent robotic followers with the money saved from averting these procedures.

Robodoc and its cousins are far more numerous in Europe than in the United States. Among the British projects in progress are use of telerobotics for pedicle screw insertion into the spine and transurethral prostate resections. At the Department of Neurology at the University of Grenoble in France, surgeons use robots to remove tumors and drain cranial fluid from patients.

Robotics projects of the Swiss Federal Institute of Technology in Lausanne, Switzerland hint at the next generation of changes, when improved robots will be more complex and have extended memory capacities, rather than simply being assigned a singular task. The Institute's Microengineering Department, which collaborates on some advanced robotics projects with NASA, has developed one such robot. It can remove a piece of scalp, switch tools when it detects a change in resistance, then proceed to the next task of draining fluid from the brain. Other research at the Institute applies robotics to the delicate task of implanting live cells. These cells produce the active substance that is then directly administered to the site to be treated. Their placement requires extraordinary accuracy—a task custom-made for a new and improved robot.

The more delicate the task, the more dexterity, tactile sensation and force feedback to the operator's hand come into play. In the United States, Dr. Stephen Jacobsen of the University of Utah in Salt Lake City developed a dextrous robotic hand that can be manipulated to screw in a light bulb without breaking it. Jacobsen has demonstrated that such a robot can be controlled remotely through multisensory input. The operator inserts an arm and hand into the master device, then manipulates the distant robotic arm into performing precision tasks. To telemedicine, this is one of several breakthroughs that mean "remote surgery" is moving closer to including remote consultation, remote diagnosis and remote training as integral parts of the health care of the future.

As the Digital Age of the 1990s dawned, technology started catching up with necessity and imagination on several levels. While the futuristic work in genetic mapping, robotics and imaging were getting underway, basic telemedicine systems also became more affordable. This was made possible by a convergence of powerful, commercially available "off-the-shelf" computing, communications and imaging technologies.

Supported by advances in wired and wireless communication, digital photography and more, health-care practitioners in the next few years will make real the possibility of delivering health care at a distance around the globe.

8

Telemedicine on the Battlefield

Mogadishu is a remote and despicable place. . . . It was like sending our soldiers to a garbage pit with a hospital.

Lt. Gen. Alcide M. LaNoue
38th Surgeon General of the U.S. Army

Fine sand, fleas, spitting cobras, three kinds of malaria, desperate hunger and drug addicts armed with AK 47s: Welcome to Operation Restore Hope. Five years ago, the paved streets of Mogadishu hosted cars and commerce. Now, buried under sand drifts, they are the home of camels and sniper fire.

The university that housed one of the premiere medical schools in Africa is riddled with bullets. In rooms where some of the brightest minds on the continent taught biochemistry and anatomy, disconsolate people now sleep and urinate. Here, as in most of the white-washed buildings with beautiful marble floors, there is no electricity or running water. Vandals have stripped out every copper wire, every pipe—anything worth anything.

What was once the Mogadishu hospital is now just filthy rooms where the sick and injured rest. No one works there on weekends, when family members administer most patient care. This is better than it was. Before United Nations soldiers cleaned up the building, exposing themselves to a plethora of nasty parasites, the hospital had even more primitive facilities.

"If you go away from civilization as far as possible, you wind up in Somalia," said one soldier. No one is safe there. Even those who tried to literally heal the country's wounds.

One of the people who came to heal the people of Somalia was Maj. Ronald Poropatich, pulmonary and critical care physician at Walter Reed Army Medical Center. He had never faced combat before. On February 20, 1993 at 8 A.M., he disembarked from a United States Army transport plane at the Mogadishu airport after a twenty-four hour flight that began in Dover, Delaware. Heat emanated from the tarmac. For the first few minutes, he watched a flurry of military personnel moving equipment, loading and unloading planes, landing Black Hawk helicopters and clutching automatic weapons.

His one-week assignment was to train his fellow doctors on the telemedicine system and find as many medical applications for it as possible. Dr. Poropatich was accompanied by Sgt. Carl Boocks, a specialist in graphics and photography, and Maj. J.B. Crowther, Information Management Officer in the Office of the Surgeon General of the Army. The portable system in the bags they carried on the plane included a laptop computer, a digital camera, a small satellite transceiver and some cables.

Doctor Poropatich's introduction to battle wounds came quickly. An Australian who had been shot the week before was nearby, relating his brush with death to fellow troops. A round had deflected off a metal piece of equipment on his uniform and went into his shoulder instead of his chest. "I'm standing there hearing him explain his story, and suddenly I realized a lot of guys are getting shot. It was a very important time for me to appreciate the danger of the situation," the doctor recalled.

Poropatich, Crowther and Boocks surveyed the airfield. Flags of Italy, Australia, Pakistan, the United Kingdom, Nigeria and the United States broadcast the United Nations' presence. The volume of military equipment and concentration of armed troops verified that the United Nations' mission involved more than just the distribution of food.

Once they left the airfield and loaded their gear onto trucks, they drove down a dusty road that paralleled the runway. Clouds of fine sand hit them as they rumbled the short distance to the 86th Evacuation Hospital. Clearly, there was a reason why the troops wore goggles.

There were Somali buildings within one hundred yards of the airfield. With or without combat experience, it became immediately evident to the doctor that even a bad shot could hit the hospital from there. United Nations troops, at this time Nigerians, were spaced every one hundred yards to protect medical personnel from the Somali threat. After a tense, hot day of standing guard, the Nigerian soldiers would return to their nearby makeshift shelters—some just cardboard boxes.

In contrast to the bursts of violence and troop activity, the Indian Ocean on the other side of the airfield offered a view of serenity. Even so, the sight of a massive United States Navy desalinization ship served as a reminder of military presence.

Seeing the hospital, Dr. Poropatich and his colleagues were struck by its proximity to the air traffic. Positioned only sixty yards from the runway, hospital staff routinely plugged their ears to dampen the high-pitched scream of C-5As. The planes were the main reason why no one got much sleep.

The hospital had been up and running since January 10, twenty-three days after the first United States troops arrived in Mogadishu. An impressive design called DEPMEDS (Deployable Medical System) was installed—five acres of interconnected canvas tents, insulated with two layers of fabric. Equipped with its own power generators, the hospital defied the Somali heat with air conditioning pumped through huge bladders hanging from the ceiling. The 104-bed facility even had nearly dust-free plastic floors. Complementing the network of tents were boxcar-sized sheds housing labs and operating rooms.

An evacuation hospital such as this one, assembled by the 86th out of Fort Campbell, Kentucky, represents the highest echelon of battlefield care. The smallest medical facility is a forward aid station, staffed by someone perhaps a year out of medical school. After stabilizing a patient there, the doctor might order the person moved to a MASH, or Mobile Army Surgical Hospital, probably the most well-known unit because of the hit television series "M*A*S*H." Lacking any major air support, a MASH might get the patient a helicopter ride to an airport for evacuation to a larger facility. Beyond the MASH is the Combat Support Hospital (CSH, pronounced "cash"), then the evacuation hospital. At each level of care, there are more physicians and more capabilities. The next stop after an "evac hospital" is a place like Landstuhl Army Regional Medical Center in Germany. If Landstuhl can't handle the case, the patient goes to Walter Reed or one of seven other major Army medical centers in the United States.

On first seeing the 86th Evacuation Hospital, Sgt. Boocks found the complex amazing: "It's the best hospital in

Mogadishu right now, the most capable medical facility in the entire country, and think of it—it's nothing more than some canvas tenting and a couple of metal trailers."

The truck carrying the telemedicine team stopped at their quarters. As in "M*A*S*H," the doctors slept in a tent labeled "The Swamp." Ropes and strings sagging with drying clothes laced the inside. Some had dressed their area with a plywood floor, others rested their cots on the sand. Everyone used mosquito nets.

Fueled by adrenaline, Poropatich overcame jet lag and met the other doctors at the daily 7:30 A.M. meeting: "I felt compelled as a physician to show up for morning report to show the docs I could hang in there with them. And I wanted to hear what kind of cases were being seen in the hospital to find out how to best use the system." One look at the assembled physicians told him, "Not too many gray-hairs." Of the eighteen doctors on site, ten had less than one year of experience in their specialty—a fact that underlined the value of the telemedicine system in Somalia.

As a fellow clinician, Poropatich felt that the doctors trusted his optimism that the new technology could put them in touch with colleagues and resources back home. Through personal training, the same emphasis on doctor-to-doctor communication that inspired the system made it welcome in the field.

Crowther and Broocks soon brought the telemedicine unit on line. Lacking any communications infrastructure—Somali warlords had ripped out phone lines throughout Mogadishu—they used the International Maritime Satellite Organization (Inmarsat) spacecraft. Tactical and administrative information, as well as medical, had to travel via satellite both within and outside of the theater of conflict.

After some initial training sessions, two doctors displayed special affinity for the computer and camera. Maj. Tom Moore had rotated through vascular surgery at Walter Reed, where Lt. Col. Ed Gomez, Chief of Peripheral Vascular Surgery and lead clinician on telemedicine, had thrust him in front of Apple technology. For Moore, the Macintosh PowerBook 180 used in the system was like an old friend—with a facelift. Complementing him on camera was Maj. Mike Hotard, a fellow general surgeon who was often armed with his own 35mm Nikon. The Kodak camera, which integrated Nikon elements, felt comfortable.

Although charged with operating the telemedicine system, the doctors were not expected to download images from the camera to the computer, compress and send them back to Walter Reed and maintain the technology. This support came from Capt. Gordon "Gordy" Murray, the Information Management Officer deployed to the 86th from Walter Reed. With the addition of Capt. Steve Allen, a radiologist, and pathologist Lt. Col. Larry Godfrey—who eventually served three tours of duty in Somalia—the field hospital telemedicine team took shape. Enthusiasm for the new system spread through the 86th.

The first image Capt. Murray sent back to Walter Reed told a story greater than a head wound. Hit accidentally by an American truck, a Somali boy had sustained a deep gash to his scalp, as well as a broken arm and leg. Attended by a neurosurgeon and two orthopedic doctors, the boy had superb care. Poropatich slipped behind them to capture an image—not for consultative or diagnostic purposes, but merely to document the event.

How sad that this child, probably running after sympathetic United States troops to claim a handout, ran into a five-ton truck storming down the road at forty-five miles per hour. Tragic. Regrettable. Common. The shocking photograph showed this to be a frequent occurrence.

In the event an action by United Nations forces injured a Somali, they were obligated to treat and rehabilitate the victim. After a marked improvement, the patient would be transferred to the Somali hospital for further convalescence. If the victim died, however, the family might be eligible for a "solatia payment," which seemed more desirable than another living relative for some families. Poropatich recalls:

> The terrible stories you would hear are that the children were thrown in front of trucks by their families, that children already dead from starvation were thrown in front of the trucks so families could collect payment.

The form of remuneration to the Somali people reflected a long-standing Muslim tradition called "diyah" (also "dia"), or blood money. Originally, it entailed trading a life for a life. The victim's family might be compensated by a certain number of camels. For example, certain Somalis would value a male at a hundred camels and a female at fifty. In modern times, within the context of "solatia payments," families might receive the appropriate number of camels or the cash equivalent.

Later, Poropatich again photographed a Somali child hit by a truck. This time it was a seven-year-old boy whose leg wound resisted treatment. The doctors who viewed the damage thought it so severe that the child would lose his foot. While watching and waiting for a change in status, nurses lifted his spirits by making balloon toys out of surgical gloves.

The image dispatched to Walter Reed in this case involved genuine consultative need. On February 23 at 4:23 A.M. E.S.T.,

Poropatich transmitted the image of a grossly infected foot along with an immediate request for a plastic surgery consultation. Data sent included the following:

Problem:	Crush injury to left foot with nonhealing wound.
History:	Five-ton truck ran over foot on 1-22-93. Emergent surgery then included repair of dorsalis pedis artery and split thickness skin graft to foot. Only part of graft on dorsum above metatarsals survived. Wound also superficially infected.
Physical Exam:	Vascular intact distally. Neuro intact. Moves toes moderately well. Wound over dorsum with nonhealing ulcers.
Laboratory:	n/a
X-ray Reports:	Fractures of metatarsals #1, 2, 3.
Clinical Images:	Left foot nonhealing wound—two photos.
Current Rx:	Daily wound dressing changes.
Specific Questions:	Should patient undergo repeat split thickness skin graft vs. crossed leg skin graft vs. amputation?

The surgeon's eyes that saw the wound 7,900 miles away at Walter Reed helped field doctors avert amputation of the boy's foot.

While saving lives clearly gave the doctors and nurses of the 86th great satisfaction, their use of telemedicine to avoid unnecessary air evacuations also pleased Central Command—and gave taxpayers a morale boost. At the rate of $7,000 per hour to operate a C-141, a twelve-hour flight to Landstuhl ran $84,000. If an empty plane returned to Mogadishu, that added another $84,000 to the price tag. Compounding that cost was the loss of a soldier brought into the field with special expertise, with a particular job to do. Finally, if the patient's condition warranted constant attention by a physician, one more highly trained professional was gone, with no replacement.

In two instances, Poropatich had strong suspicions about pending air evacuations and sent images to Washington. One requested a consultation; the other broke new ground by requiring a diagnosis.

The picture transmitted to Walter Reed on February 24, 1993 showed skin lesions on the right side of a soldier's abdomen. Field doctors had appropriately diagnosed his condition as chronic angio edema, an unusual hereditary problem producing little rashes or eruptions about the size of a quarter. Aware that such rashes can invade airways to create great difficulty breathing, attending physicians called for air evacuation. The patient's history accompanied the image sent to the Chief of Allergy at Walter Reed, who concluded correctly that the skin lesions, confined to the skin, posed no danger to him.

Fortunately, the transmission exchange with Walter Reed took only about an hour. The soldier returned to duty as the hospital came under threat of attack around 10 P.M. Lights went out. Staff rushed back to their tents to put on flak jackets and helmets or "steel pots." Gunshots frightened hospital personnel as they pushed barricades into place on the perimeter of the hospital. Weapons were issued to those who knew how to use them.

The uproar occurred on a Wednesday night during Ramadan, a period during which all faithful Muslims must fast between dawn and dusk, riots choked the city. Somalis killed each other. United Nations soldiers came under repeated attack.

The 86th Evacuation Hospital's proximity to the Somali people made it easy for unfriendly locals to lob grenades into the hospital compound. Would it happen? Would bands of Somalis overrun the little outposts controlled by Nigerians? Not knowing the degree of involvement by Somali people, the entire complex went to alert status. The hospital survived; Poropatich went back to smoking cigarettes.

Ugly bumps around a young soldier's eyes alarmed the hospital ophthalmologist. He feared systemic lupus erythematosus, an auto-immune disease causing red lesions to form on the face and scalp. The soldier's evacuation seemed imminent. Seeking expertise from the dermatology department at Walter Reed, Poropatich sent images back home. In this case, they had a clear diagnostic value. It was discovered that the patient suffered from contact dermatitis, not lupus. Quickly, doctors determined that he had an allergy to the rubber in the goggles that protected his eyes from the gusts of fine sand.

While the value of image transmission clearly enhanced the performance and confidence of the 86th, having a direct link to a medical center's data also yielded improved health care. The issue of using the drug "Mefloquine" emerged when some troops suspected they were pregnant. Active duty soldiers in Somalia received the drug, used to prevent malaria, on a weekly basis. Questions arose: Were suspicions correct that it caused damage to a fetus? What data were available on the use of Mefloquine during pregnancy? Instead of guessing or hoping, soldiers could review studies extracted by a MEDLINE (database) search, courtesy of Walter Reed. Most concluded that the clear benefit of fending off a malaria parasite outweighed the unproven risk of taking the drug.

Sensitive political issues surrounded another case in which telemedicine focused on a dead Somali and the soldier who shot him. When met Lt. Col. Larry Godfrey, he was reading

Guns and Ammo. Assigned to the 86th because of a forensic investigation, the pathologist had to determine whether a particular NATO round, illegal in the hands of Army personnel, had killed a Somali civilian. No one doubted that the soldier's life was in jeopardy and he had a right to shoot. The issue was whether or not he used an "illegal" round to do it. Ironically, use of this type of round was approved for other United Nations forces, including the Marines. Not so for United States Army soldiers.

Dr. Godfrey saw an immediate application for the telemedicine technology. He and Poropatich sent pictures of the point of entry and the round, juxtaposed with other objects to show precise size, to the Armed Forces Institute of Pathology (AFIP). The clarity of the images helped the experts reach a verdict: There was no wrongdoing on the American soldier's part. Although Godfrey carried unusual credentials for this investigation—a small arms expert, he is known for living military life with gusto—the telemedicine system brought the power of AFIP to the final decision.

Forensic pathology cases like the one that first brought Godfrey to Mogadishu are not common fare at evacuation hospitals. Under normal circumstances, a pathologist would not be assigned to a battlefield unit. Interpretation of blood smears and other microscopic samples might fall to the lab officer; before entering medical school, that was Poropatich's job.

Here is a probable scenario: A junior Medical Corps officer who went through a one-year course in laboratory medicine may be the one closest to the smear, but may not feel comfortable calling something malaria. Similarly, the technician may have real problems determining what kind of infection lives in the pus coming from a soldier's wound. Poropatich hoped that he could hook up the telemedicine system to a microscope to offer a new way of assessing a pathology diagnosis made in the field.

Unfortunately, he lacked the metal adapter that could link the microscope and the camera. He looked around the tent hospital asking himself the frustrating question, "What do I need?" He decided he needed something that could form a seal at the camera lens and block all ambient light from there to the microscope. Any intrusion of light would compromise the quality of the image coming into the camera. It was an oddly simple solution; a styrofoam coffee cup joined the gadgets in the Army's mobile telemedicine system. "The cup was beveled so I could just keep cutting off parts of it until I had a good seal with the diameter of the camera lens itself," said Poropatich. I went through five cups until I got one that had a good seal."

He and Boocks took the sculpted cup and hooked it up to a microscope. By positioning a camera on top of the cup, while one person manipulated the camera and one focused the microscope, they were able to bring up an image onto the camera that was, as Poropatich admits, "somewhat in focus." The photo they generated and transmitted to Walter Reed showed red blood cells, with a large purple body on top of one of them. They had succeeded in recording a discernible image of a malaria parasite.

On the receiving end at Walter Reed, Dr. Gomez and Fred Copeman, the biomedical engineer in charge of the technology at Walter Reed, cheered the demonstration of photo microscopy with the telemedicine system. In an important way, this diagnostic-quality image validated the choice they had advocated of affordable off-the-shelf technology, rather than the costly alternatives that had been proposed.

In the field, this victory offered inspiration. If it could work in diagnosis, a similar configuration could be used in ophthalmology by attaching the camera to the slit lamp used in eye exams. This time, parts were ordered.

Their mission completed, Poropatich, Crowther and Boocks let two armed guards usher them to the transport plane that would carry them home. They had high hopes that the field team would actually use the telemedicine system, and were not disappointed.

Greeting them at Walter Reed was the image of a soldier who had sustained a shrapnel wound to the face. The metal fragment had sliced across the outer lining of the eye and came to rest where the nose and eye meet—the "canthus" of the eye. An image sent over the network was indisputable evidence of a an information bridge between the 86th and Walter Reed Hospital.

More than a technological victory, it also brought the field doctors much needed help. The staff ophthalmologist for the 86th had just departed for Landstuhl to take his boards. Without his expertise, uncertainty about whether or not to remove the fragment on-site plagued the doctors. Walter Reed ruled, "Don't touch it. Air evac him. "

"Doctors take pictures of patients anyway," Moore observed. "We have them to train medical students, put in the patient's file, for textbooks, for journals. That's why the telemed system isn't intrusive."

Images continued to come, some of them taken by Murray of the hospital itself, the airfield, the gutted Somali buildings. Moore slipped in a couple that showed a fairly common sight, too: the opened belly of a Somali whose intestinal tract housed several large worms.

Moore summed up the reaction of the 86th to the location:

I think every bush in Somalia has thorns. Every insect bites. Every snake is poisonous. We thought we probably never should have gone there, but we were proud to do some good.

9

Rescue 2000

Within a decade, I think we're really going to come to the Dick Tracy watch, which will probably sell on the commercial market for about one hundred dollars.

Col. Richard M. Satava, MD
United States Advanced Research Projects Agency

What if Operation Restore Hope were to occur in the year 2000 instead of having occurred in 1992? What will happen to people involved in a hurricane, car accident or other traumatic incident in the future?

Trauma means immediacy in patient care. It requires a new model for telemedicine. NASA's early work in biotelemetry, in improving both equipment and communications protocols used in projects such as STARPAHC, influenced the development of advanced care ambulances. This mobile capability is central to a telemedicine system designed for emergency care. The use of the Army's portable unit, deployed in Mogadishu, Zagreb and Macedonia in 1993, also suggests the kind of field system that can help save lives in the "golden hour," that first hour after a serious injury when the immediacy of treatment means life or death.

Installing a telemedicine system in the emergency department of a hospital supports its staff in handling complex trauma cases, but the real challenge is not in this locale. It is in the place where the person was injured—on a highway, on a battlefield or in a country church collapsed by a hurricane.

In America, for instance, the United States Department of Defense has startling statistics about battlefield casualties that underline the need to bring advanced care to the site of the injury. Of the American soldiers who die from battlefield injuries, about 90 percent are dead by the time they reach the MASH unit or other definitive care facility. Since World War I, this mortality rate has remained relatively constant. On the other hand, there has been a dramatic reduction in the death rate for soldiers who survived the trip to the hospital.

In an effort to move the highest level of medical expertise to the wounded soldier, Col. Richard M. Satava, MD, research head of Advanced Biomedical Technology at the United States Advanced Research Projects Agency is directing joint military-civilian efforts at developing technologies for "the modern meical battlefield." Costs of related research and development projects around the world are often shouldered by the American government. Some of the work emanates from the Technology Reinvestment Program, aimed at getting dual-use technologies from the military into the civilian world.

The first demonstration of these futuristic devices and systems occurred on June 28, 1993 at Fort Gordon, Georgia. It opened eyes in the world of emergency medicine about what the future holds for an injured patient.

Every soldier wears the Personal Status Monitor (PSM), which Satava calls "the Dick Tracy watch." The four components of this computer-on-a-wristband provide information on vital signs, location, "friend or foe" status and medical history. A host of miniature, non-invasive sensors monitor blood pressure, pulse, heartbeat and oxygen saturation.

For example, say a soldier takes a bullet. The soldier's watch detects a shift in vital signs. An encrypted position locator relying on the satellite-based Global Positioning System is triggered and alerts the local unit and command of the wounded soldier's location within three meters. On a computer screen in the MASH tent, a soldier monitoring the grid of the battlefield sees where the victim is and dispatches aid. If it's a serious trauma, two medics equipped with advanced resuscitation gear race to the position. As help moves toward the site, the "friend or foe" identification signal emitted by everyone's PSM averts "shoot first, ask questions later" mistakes. Arriving at the site, one medic removes the fourth component from the PSM, an electronic dog tag.

Similar in concept to the Woodward-Kaufman meditag described earlier, the tag slips into a hand-held computer and communications device designed to guide emergency medical care by reading the tag and transmitting critical data. Quickly, physicians at the MASH know the soldier's identification, medical history and current condition. They work with the medic at the victim's side to determine the best next step. Real-time video permits the physician to see exactly what the medic sees, answer questions immediately and guide the medic through the first seconds and minutes of care. This "telementoring" relationship is not meant to intrude upon the medic's role, but to apply specific expertise if it's needed.

Two complementary options for intensive care exist at this point. If it has been determined that the soldier can be stabilized and safely transported some distance without surgery, the medics will place the victim in a high technology incubator with as much life-saving support as a modern emergency room. If the soldier requires immediate surgery, a MASH physician will perform the surgery—remotely—after the soldier is transported to a nearby station or truck in the field.

It sounds as though these options are visions of a science fiction writer. In fact, they are real in today's scientific world. Now in the advanced prototype stage, they are within reach of today's military and civilian emergency medical teams.

The incubator's original name, "Trauma Pod," was dropped so it wouldn't sound like a threat from outer space. Project head Col. Bill Wiessman, MD, of Walter Reed Army Medical Center, has renamed the protective environment LSTAT, for Life Support for Trauma and Transfer. He was also gravely concerned that early models resembled coffins and body bags, so LSTAT now resembles a small, transparent tent.

Ahead of schedule, Wiessman and his civilian partner, Sarcos Corporation of Salt Lake City, Utah have readied LSTAT for civilian and military service in 1995. One reason for the accelerated progress is the rate at which critical technological developments occurred in fields such as microminiaturized electronics, advanced computer algorithms for sensing and monitoring, flat panel data displays, wireless communications networks and more.

Conceptually, the LSTAT builds on the decades-old incubator, but is more like a portable modern emergency room. It is a five-layer carrier, 18 inches high and weighing not quite 100 pounds in order to accommodate space and weight restrictions in helicopters and other emergency conveyances. A pan on the bottom provides stability. The Kevlar-covered sled of sensors, communications tools and other life support aids rests on the base; it accommodates the stretcher bearing the patient. A windowed protective cover rests on a frame over an unconscious patient and is sealed at the sides to create a weatherproof and temperature-controlled environment. Conscious patients are usually transported without the cover since they have a greater ability to maintain their body temperature.

A guiding principle of LSTAT is "closed-loop" health care, clinically proven and advanced in the United States by LDS Hospital in Salt Lake City, Utah. A closed loop system sends a signal to a computer, the computer makes a decision about therapy, then institutes the therapy. The therapy can be a number of things—an intravenous solution, oxygen or drug. Among other systems, LDS has all respirators on a closed-loop, central, computerized control. Minute-to-minute monitoring of patients on respirators has not only improved the quality of care that patients have received, but it has also reduced costs and improved the rate at which LDS doctors wean patients off the respirators. In fact, soon after LDS introduced the closed-loop approach in the mid-1980s, the hospital saw annual savings in the millions. Such systems can be overridden, but almost never are, because therapeutic decisions based on real-time data have far greater value than those based on historical data.

Closed-loop control has distinct applications for monitoring patients with chronic conditions, as well as trauma cases. In the case of diabetes, a glucose sensor can control the amount of insulin provided. Similarly, with anesthesia delivery, it is very difficult for a nurse or doctor to control the flow because of all the parameters involved. A human being simply can't make the required changes in the same time a computer can make them.

A corollary application of the closed-loop system is monitoring patients remotely—in their homes, for example. Wiessman's partnership program with Stanford University involves using the Army's remote monitors to keep tabs on seriously ill patients who have been discharged from the university hospital. This is a variation on the prototype home system now in place in test sites around Augusta, Georgia.

Ordinary wired and wireless phone networks host the data flow on blood pressure, pulse, heartbeat, chest fluid level, weight and other physiological signs. Independent of the physician, readings will be tracked, recorded and interpreted. If the patient experiences any meaningful change, the computer will identify that patient and alert the medical staff. It is designed to improve the quality of health care for chronically ill patients and to cut the cost of their health care.

Some might envision a home-bound grandparent wrapped in wire to accomplish this feat. In fact, the project involves "weaving" sensors into fabric and relying on light, wearable devices like a wristwatch embedded with the Global Positioning System to give precise locations. It might be considered the civilian version of the PSM.

Back on the battlefield, the medic transfers the patient to the carrier and intubates the patient to keep the airway open. The carrier, with its integrated computer system providing closed loop care, is then moved to the hospital. In the meantime, data on the patient's status is constantly transmitted from the carrier to the hospital. A miniature respirator on the bottom of the unit, an oxygen supply (replenished by reprocessing external air), a number of monitors, temperature control environmental regulators, filters to protect against biological or chemical contamination, a stable bullet-proof platform—all these things and more combine to keep the patient alive during the golden hour.

When a bullet wound is life-threatening, the victim cannot wait past the golden hour for surgery. Therefore, the surgeon must electronically come to the patient in the field. The injured soldier is carried to a specially equipped truck. Medics prepare the patient for emergency surgery, then move a light, suspended robotic device and cameras into place near the operating table. A physician at the MASH unit can now operate immediately.

This technical achievement, called telepresence surgery, involves the completely believable illusion that doctor and patient are in close proximity when they may actually be separated by miles. Dr. Philip S. Green, Director of the Biomedical Engineering Research Laboratory at Stanford Research Institute (SRI International) and president of the offshoot Telesurgical Corporation, is refining a system that, even in its early form, has fooled physicians and surgical residents into thinking they were working on something right in front of them.

This is not a virtual-reality technology, however. The image that is seen *is* real and the surgeon's actions result in a *real* effect. Again, the difference is that the slicing, sewing or snipping that appears to be happening in front of the surgeon is actually happening elsewhere. When the technique was demonstrated at Fort Gordon in 1993, a surgeon at a portable workstation one hundred feet away from the surgical site, where a nurse assisted him, successfully performed a procedure on a pig.

The telepresence surgeon goes to work at a console. With the help of a light pair of polarized glasses and a stereoscopic cathode ray tube, the view on the table is one of a completely realistic world—like looking through a very clean plate of glass with objects beneath it. There is no sense that the "work area" is really a mirror with two images that the glasses organize for the brain. The surgical instrument feels real and moves in a predictable and natural way. In telepresence, the human being controls the robot at a remote site. Three-dimensional vision, stereophonic sound, tactile sensations and force feedback satisfy the brain's desire for a complete sensory experience. Very simply, it is a two-part system with the operative site and the surgical workstation.

At the operative site, a pair of video cameras mounted above the surgical area at the proper distance and angle permit transmission of stereoscopic vision. The cameras can be either analog or digital; even the thumb-sized variety of digital camera could be used. Six surgical lamps are attached to the vertical bars of the camera mount. Two microphones, cradled in something as soft and shock absorbent as foam rubber, rest near the site to provide stereophonic sound. Of all the elements, the most complicated is the remote manipulator—and this could be a scalpel, forceps, hemostat or other tool—with five axes of movement, force feedback and tactile feedback (that is, the normal senses of pressure and motion). Running up its back are multi-colored lines. Finally, the whole ensemble runs on an off-the-shelf high-end personal computer.

Experiments with the system have demonstrated an amazing degree of dexterity. The remotely manipulated scalpel can slice a grape into one-millimeter sections, precisely touch the head of a pin at least twenty-five consecutive times and perform simple dissection on a pig kidney. Forceps allow the operator to thread tiny beads on a thin wire.

"I actually get fooled on this," admits Dr. Green, a modest, white-haired visionary who has more experience with telepresence than anyone else. "Just today when I was setting it up, some of the pieces were out of visual range (at the surgical workstation), and I automatically reached in with my hand to place them where they belonged." Of course, he got a fistful of air.

From a patient's perspective, the thought of a robotic device performing an invasive procedure at the direction of a remote surgeon may seem frightening, or at least undesirable. The potential of telepresence surgery , however, involves inherent features that actually improve surgical technique. On a basic level, an electronic instrument stabilized in a workstation can be programmed to filter out the tremor of a surgeon's hand. With the introduction of three-dimensional imaging techniques allowing for maps of the precise surgical site, the system could also be programmed to prevent accidental variances from the intended procedure.

Dr. Green designed the telepresence system to improve on laparoscopic surgery, but it was quickly evident that solving the visual and tactile problems of doing laparoscopic surgery also made remote surgery possible. Instead of a long cut, giving the surgeon an open view of the problem, laparoscopy involves a small cut. A tiny camera inserted into the area helps the surgeon make the correction in a minimally invasive way. Unfortunately, it's also completely counterintuitive. A sort of house of mirrors for the surgeon, laparoscopy imposes a reversed view of the surgical site and causes depth perception problems and disorientation with the instrument. Currently, conducting laparoscopic surgery requires special training and particular skill beyond standard surgical technique. It forces the surgeon to adapt to a technology, rather than the technology accommodating the surgeon.

In order for a patient to reap the benefits of this minimally invasive technique, which includes the advantages of reduced recovery time and minimal scarring, the surgeon has to look at a television screen, while one hand is on an instrument that is working inside a damaged knee, for example. Every motion is made in the wrong motion, in the sense that there is no natural hand-eye coordination, and a little movement makes a lot of difference.

Telepresence restores the feeling of performing an open surgery; it delivers dexterity. It is astonishing how easily and quickly a laparoscopy can be performed with the system—a fact that should save countless hours of operating room and professional time. Some surgeons never learned the laparoscopic technique, so their ability to convert open surgeries to laparoscopic ones with telepresence will also save money as well as reduce patient suffering, hospitalization and time away from activities. These factors will drive the commercial viability of the system and advance the probability of its application to remote surgery of all kinds, including remote laparoscopies. Telepresence technology will become practical before the year 2000.

In an ideal world, the wounded soldier would be transported back to the MASH unit for post-operative care, with a telemedicine link to the staff of a major medical center keeping their expertise flowing to the recovering soldier. Similarly, if remote surgery were done on a French farmer whose truck overturned on him in the field, the patient would be moved to the nearest hospital for continuing care with the help of distant specialists.

Two things need to be said about this ideal world. First, the ability to put physical expertise, as well as image and text data, at the injury site is predicated on the existence of a geographically comprehensive, high performance communications network—an "information superhighway," in the current American political vernacular. Secondly, in the real world, the hardware/software cost of having such comprehensive trauma care around the globe is, to say the least, a significant inhibitor.

There must be intermediate steps to improve trauma care while more sophisticated technologies are moved into place, networks continue to evolve and costs are lowered. The Army's portable, low-cost system that went to Somalia surfaces as a problem-solving model. Advances in hand-held computing devices offer some hope that trauma care can be improved with affordable, off-the-shelf technology.

Vigorous competition in the mobile computing world has yielded commercial devices that extend the possibility for telemedicine consultations beyond the walls of a hospital, a clinic or even a home. For instance, the United States Army put a portable system into the battlefield. In the spring of 1993, television in many countries covered this feat. In contrast, there are now shelves of mobile computers that offer some level of imaging and communications capabilities in a single unit. One weighs five pounds and can be carried or attached to a docking station in an ambulance, police car or fire engine. It's essentially a smart, empty box into which three small modules can be docked—a digital camera, cellular telephone or personal communicator, a CD-ROM carrying a medical library, a small printer and so on. With what is called a TelePad 3, a police officer arriving on an accident scene could say, "crushed ribs" and immediately see the prescribed emergency care on the computer screen. A record of the rescue could also be made orally; the officer could sign it and the whole file could be transmitted to a hospital before the patient even arrived. In this way, a roughly five-pound, $5,000 machine could serve as the most basic portable telemedicine system—a field unit of the network—that could interface with the more advanced telemedicine equipment at a hospital.

In the near future, an ambulance arriving at an accident scene might also have a portable direct digital imager, a small filmless X-ray machine that can transmit images from the field to the specialist. It would be a kind of miniature cousin of the digital mammography machine.

Expected to emerge from the Advanced Research Project Agency's labs in 1995, this cigar-box sized piece of equipment will look like an ordinary X-ray cassette of 1994, but it will be a hundred times more sensitive than current systems. The cassette, in standard X-ray systems, is what holds the film; in this case it holds the digital receptor. As a corollary, this means it will use 1/100 the amount of power for the same amount of X-rays taken today. The medic or emergency medical technician will slip the cassette under the patient and take the picture. The device exposes the plate. The plate then automatically acquires the image, compresses it and transmits it to another room, a MASH unit or a hospital.

Direct digital imaging adds another dimension of reliability to remote care. Whoever took the picture would not have to wait for a radiologist to check it to make sure it was shot correctly. Unless the doctor, nurse or medic had a complete mental lapse and shot the wrong body part, patient care would not be delayed because of having to reshoot an X-ray. The digital imager automatically corrects for exposure by changing the "dynamic range."

If, for example, there were too much white in the picture, the computer could be reset to render a contrast that's exactly right for the area under scrutiny. If a liver were pictured, the practitioner, as well as the remote physician who is providing diagnostic input, would see the shape, colorations, veins and arteries of the liver just as if the image were captured perfectly.

All of these mobile, powerful and, in many cases, relatively low-cost devices mean an immediate transformation of the way emergency medical teams can serve victims of trauma—and get them successfully through the golden hour.

No matter how good the technology, however, the future of emergency medicine is only bright if training techniques keep moving forward. This is where virtual reality enters the picture in a powerful way. Virtual reality is a computer science that constructs intangible three-dimensional worlds that seem real through the stimulation of multiple senses. For physicians facing trauma cases, the same workstation used for real-time telepresence surgery could conceivably be switched over to a training mode to become a surgical simulator. A surgeon potentially confronting many types of wounds could then simulate injuries and practice on a computer-generated, three-dimensional abdomen with organs and surgical instruments. Similar training programs could be developed for medics and other emergency medicine practitioners to sharpen their skills in handling a full spectrum of injuries.

10

On the Road to the Future

The advent of powerful neural computer technology, combined with artificial intelligence systems and high speed telecommunications, provides the opportunity for the practice of medicine to change from isolated individual encounters to an integrated national and international medical system.

Bernard L. Crowe
Australian Institute of Health and Welfare

When Norway sanctioned telemedicine as a new and exciting adjunct to face-to-face care, it wasn't long before other nations followed suit. Singapore's aggressive use of advanced communications systems will make telemedicine an instant reality there, too. Meanwhile, in some other countries where the government manages health care, there have been delays and pitfalls in implementing extensive telemedicine programs. To a great extent, success depends on where health care falls in the scheme of national priorities, and how efficiently nations can deal with technical issues.

In Europe, a force driving telemedicine forward consists of two programs under the direction of the European Community. In both the Advanced Informatics in Medicine (AIM) and Research and Development in Advanced Communication in Europe (RACE) programs, a combination of research groups, medical institutions and industry are looking at health care applications of information technology. In TELEMED, a project of RACE, the goal is to find the technical problems in teleconsultation. Once these are framed, it is easier to develop a set of technical specifications regarding telemedicine system equipment.

In the United States, free market concerns drive health care delivery systems more than human need does. Therefore, it will take a very strong political will, coupled with the co-operation of big business, to make telemedicine happen on a large-scale basis. One instance where it *has* happened, but on a small scale, was in the state of Georgia. This state's political leadership has teamed with business, academia and the communities in a mission to improve health care for all citizens. The result is a model network, centered at the Medical College of Georgia (MCG). This is a prime example of a geographically comprehensive, sustainable, multi-functional and innovative telemedicine network.

MCG opens eyes to what, because of telemedicine, the future holds when people are ill. Technically speaking, it isn't that MCG's system is the best, but that it makes the patients' quality of life better on a daily basis.

The commitment to change the status of health care in Georgia began with MCG hiring Dr. Jay Sanders. Sanders had been at Ken Bird's side during his pioneering work at Massachusetts General Hospital. In developing a design for telemedicine services in Georgia, the modest Sanders said he just did "a parallel upgrade of what Bird taught me."

During the first month of the telemedicine system's operation in Georgia, Todd Marshall, a beefy farmer, came into the examination room at the rural hospital. His complaint was that a rash covered his body. Since the attending physician at the hospital wasn't familiar with this type of problem, he used the remote consult system to call a dermatologist at the Medical College of Georgia. Standing in front of the camera, Marshall showed the doctor, who was more than one hundred miles away, his bare chest and arms. The dermatologist asked, "Todd, do you have this rash anyplace else?" Todd said, "Oh, sure, doc," then turned around, bent over and bared all. He was right—the rash *did* cover him everywhere. If it hadn't been possible for the rural hospital's physicians to utilize telemedicine to find a cure, Todd Marshall may have had that rash for the rest of his life.

In the beginning, scientists shaped the design of the telemedicine system with three major criteria in mind: open architecture, modularity and strategic redundancy. The first two help maintain flexibility in responding to changing needs of patients and new developments in technology. Redundancy ensures that maintenance of the system is transparent to users.

Since the system came to life in November 1991, shutdown has caused only one cancellation of a consultation. This wasn't due to a broken camera lens or blown computer, however; both of those could have been replaced immediately. Rather, the cancellation was because of what the telephone company unaffectionately calls a "cable finder"—to a farmer or construction worker, a backhoe. A digging accident near a country road had severed the line between MCG and Dodge County Hospital in distant Eastman, Georgia.

When a patient, like Luke Parsons, has a heart problem, consultations between MCG in Augusta, Georgia and one of the local hospitals on the network could go like this:

"Did you notice how that murmur increased in intensity when we sat the patient up?" asks the cardiologist in Augusta.

The referring physician hears the sound. "That's a classic indicator of a floppy mitral valve," the cardiologist says.

The specialist continues to co-examine Mr. Parsons, who is sitting comfortably in a room 130 miles away in the single-story Dodge County Hospital with his own family doctor. Simultaneously, the physician team checks eyes, ears, nose and throat with scopes attached to a very small camera. Together, they review chest X-rays and EKGs and view a cardiac ultrasound. This is generally done by reviewing a tape of the procedures, but it could be done live, if warranted. When the specialist sees a particular image which is meaningful, he freeze-frames it and sends the image into storage on a personal computer, where it will be examined in detail later.

After Mr. Parsons leaves, the consulting physician and the referring generalist discuss the case. Pulling up one of the stored images, the cardiologist turns to a flat plastic pad with a square marked "draw area." He uses an electronic pen to draw a circle around the aortic knob: "You know, I think there's a problem here." The family doctor says, "I see the calcification you're talking about, but I think there's also something going on in the left base of the lung." Using her control pad, she selects another color and draws an arrow toward a left lower lobe lesion: "This is what I'm concerned about."

Three weeks later, moments before the patient arrives for a follow-up exam, the two doctors prepare. Instead of opening up a chart and reading a few scribbled lines, however, they simultaneously view and hear highlights of the last session—X-rays, heartbeat, portions of the ultrasound, breathing irregularities. The specialist pulls up the chest X-ray with annotations and says, "Here. This is what I was concerned about." They could replay the entire exam if they felt it were necessary.

The scenario between the two doctors calls to mind the wise words of Dr. Bruce Houtchens, a key player in the American-Soviet Spacebridge program: "When the right people are present, the right things get done." A network like MCG's that can accomplish the transmission of clear pictures and quality audio—images and sounds from outside *and* inside the body—offers four major medical advantages. First, the patient now has access to a doctor who specializes in his or her problem. Second, the rural doctor is no longer isolated from the rest of the medical community. Third, the doctor consulting with a colleague, whether it's in the same area of specialization or a different one, receives a type of continuing medical education. Finally, the service enhances the continuity of care—the patient can stay close to home, or even in the home, during treatment.

In the event that a patient in one of the local hospitals on the network urgently needs help from a specialist, a doctor or nurse can contact MCG's . The emergency room (ER) physician in charge contacts the appropriate specialist, but immediately arranges to see the person over the system. ER staff receive special training in operating the equipment, so they can proceed with the emergency consult without help from technical staff. If they forget how to use one of the components, they can make a toll-free call to a twenty-four-hour technical assistance service.

One night, Ellen Ann Washburne, a cancer patient in a Swainsboro, Georgia clinic, took a serious downward turn. She had multiple complications, and seemed headed for renal failure. Staff at the local hospital did not know which treatment path to take, so they called MCG.

Early the next morning, three doctors at the clinic got on the network with a general surgeon and a gynecology oncologist, a specialist focused on cancer affecting the female reproductive system, at MCG. None had ever before been in their respective telemedicine rooms. One of the Swainsboro physician's put a liver scan on the view box; the problem was instantly apparent to the MCG specialist. He diagnosed the problem and mapped out a successful treatment program in ten minutes.

Primarily, Ms. Washburne needed an operation routinely done at the local hospital. If the Swainsboro doctors hadn't found that out, though, she would have been transferred to MCG, far away from her family and at a much higher cost.

Because the advent of telemedicine as opposed to traditional medical care has come so quickly, there are few giant laboratories or posh offices yet devoted to it. At MCG, the specialist sits in a small room once used to store linens. In fact, if the room needed to store linens again, the entire computer, imaging and communications system can simply be wheeled somewhere else. At the fifty-bed Hospital, for another example, the practitioner works with a counterpart system that sits unobtrusively in the emergency department. Currently their connection is made on dedicated T1 lines, that is, bundles of channels that provide the signal-carrying capacity required for real-time video transmission as well as an array of examination devices.

Not only the offices where its practitioners are found, but also some of the components of the system itself seem modest in comparison to the science-fiction stories in which similar machines were once envisioned. There are fifteen components of the system. Among them are ordinary pieces of office and home equipment: fax machine, telephone, desktop computer and video cassette (VCR) or compact disc (CD). Notes about the consultation go into an on-line database so they can be easily added to the patient's chart. At the other end, the fax machine provides auxiliary backup. After a consultation, the specialist also faxes the session notes to the referring physician. Another component of the system is a "codec," short for coder-decoder, which converts signals from analog to digital and encrypts them to protect the patient's privacy.

In this system, there are also scopes, controls, an EKG and four separate cameras. Camera One is the "patient interview camera," a standard unit found in any videoconferencing system. Before a consultation begins, MCG uses it to increase the comfort level for patients and doctors. Fifteen minutes prior to the scheduled consult, the telemedicine coordinator at each site checks out the system. At the remote site the coordinator introduces the patient to the setup, including controls for sound and camera adjustment that will be used either by the physician or by the patient. During that time, the MCG coordinator also talks with the patient so the person can get accustomed to interaction over the system.

Camera Two is more exciting and functions on another level. This camera can capture the entire exam room as well as a single hair. It is the main diagnostic unit, a color camera that also contains microprocessors like a computer. It pans, tilts and zooms to a power of sixteen. The diagnostic camera, nicknamed "camera on a stick" at MCG, is mounted on a tripod at the remote site. The tripod is perpendicular to the view box where the X-ray sits. This arrangement allows the consulting physician to zoom in to magnify the X-ray, refocus and even change contrast to see minute details, if necessary. It enables a closeness to and clarity of all or a portion of the X-ray that viewing the actual film or transmitted image of the actual film would not permit.

Camera Three is for graphics which show heart activity, such as EKGs or graphs. Mounted above a tray where the graph or film would normally rest, it also acts as a built-in backup camera. If the diagnostic camera were to fail, the document camera could substitute, zooming in and focusing on tiny detail. In fact, it captures whorls on a fingerprint so clearly that Georgia's Department of Corrections is studying special applications for it. One interesting note is that some patients have come to the consultation concerned that they had confused their medication. They then simply dropped the pills in question on the tray and the specialist has no trouble reading their tiny identifying marks.

Now the system has moved from the relatively simple to the complex, from the realistic to the futuristic. Camera Four, the first component of MCG's system to distinguish it technologically from others, is a microsoakable camera. It is a close relative of the tiny units used in laparoscopic surgery. By adding a hand-tooled adapter onto the end of this camera, it can add "eyes" to any scope—otoscope (looks inside the nose), ophthalmoscope (eyes), microscope (cells), endoscope (gastrointestinal tract) and so on. This is the kind of adapter that Dr. Poropatich needed in Somalia, when he improvised with a styrofoam cup to photograph microscopic images of the malaria parasite. Literally any scope procedure can be done live over the telemedicine system, greatly increasing the range of specialists that can do remote diagnoses. A patient's ear lesion, optic nerve, blood smears or cell samples can be magnified and photographically isolated by zooming in on them.

For example, as the scope is moving around to the eye, the specialist might spot the problem or a suspicious area and say to the referring physician, "Stop right there. Could you send that, please?" The doctor simply reaches over to a flat, touch-sensitive plastic pad and touches the area marked "Send" with an electronic pen tethered to the unit. Instantly, the isolated image appears on one of the specialist's three screens and is ready for discussion and annotation. Both doctors can draw on it in different colors, or insert text. They can save the image with or without the notes, and erase anything that is no longer useful. Another option is moving to a blank screen, or interactive white board, to facilitate a general diagrammatic discussion. A touch of this same pen on the pad will increase or lower volume, zoom in with the camera or pan, or move forward or backward through a set of slides.

With electronics at the heart of a telemedicine system, tools of a routine examination can assume a much greater diagnostic value than their unplugged cousins. One reason is that a digital signal is composed of discrete elements. Unlike an analog, or continuous, signal that can merely be played louder or softer, or made darker or lighter, a digital signal can be enhanced and manipulated. For example, in order to transmit the sounds of a patient's beating heart from a local hospital, the doctor can use an electronic stethoscope. With a simple pocket stethoscope, one beat is one sound. The new model allows the cardiac cycle to be electronically dissected, so the specialist can shut sounds off during the systolic, or contraction, phase of the heartbeat and only listen to the diastolic. With the certainty that only diastolic sounds are being heard, the physician can pinpoint which valves are potentially involved in a problem.

Another advantage of the system is that any of the images in the examination records can be sent, including single frames of the video tape. The ability to freeze a frame of the video exam record has special benefits in pediatric medicine, where a sick two-year-old may not respond to a doctor's command to "sit still."

Finally, the system provides automatic access to Scientific American Medicine Consult, SAM CD, an on-line medical literature service. If there are nuances to a diagnosis or a treatment program that the consulting specialist wants the primary care physician to know about, in addition to sending consultative notes, relevant literature can also be transmitted.

These electronic connections to mainstream medicine could signal the end of professional isolation for remote doctors. This isolation is the very thing that Dr. Pedersen cited as the reason that money, vacations and other incentives could not lure doctors to the far reaches of northern Norway. Most specialists have little or no desire to distance themselves from modern techniques and the latest research by locating their medical practice in a remote community; they stay where the intellectual action is. And doctors who do serve outlying regions may find that, even if they are doing their best, the isolation means they are using outdated therapies.

Sanders sees telemedicine as having a two-sided benefit in this context:

That there is professional isolation is quite clear. The system of medical education is ridiculous! People like myself are trained in major academic medical centers, and we become addicted to all our subspecialty colleagues and all of the high technology that's available to us. Then we cut that educational umbilical cord, and we end up in the real world. If the real world is a rural community, we have access to neither the technology nor the colleagues. That type of professional isolation is very clear.

I've spent my entire professional career in academic medicine. I have a very special type of practice here—a referral practice. I don't have to set up an office; my office is set up for me. God help me if I ever have to go out into the real world to set up a practice! I would not have the slightest idea how to do that, and if I were in a rural community, I would not have the slightest idea what my patient profile would be like. What kind of patients would I be dealing with? Yet, the irony is that I'm the one who's educating the physician who ends up in the real world.

In the areas of medical and health education, there's a close corollary to the benefits of telemedicine on doctor training. In fact, Sanders views continuing medical education as a fundamental mission of telemedicine:

We've got to make sure that access to care does not simply translate into bringing a patient to a physician, whether in person or electronically. We've got to bring the patient to a qualified and up-to-date physician.

Telemedicine only fulfills part of its potential if a specialist strides into a distant rural examining room and logs a correct diagnosis and life-saving treatment. Telemedicine provides a four-tiered process of continuing medical education for the rural physician: examination of a patient by a consulting specialist, discussion of the case, a copy of the specialists consultative notes and up-to-date medical information.

The old-fashioned way of accomplishing continuing medical education required for doctors in the United States to maintain their licenses is incredibly difficult for physicians who live in remote areas or practice alone. They have to close their practice for a week or more while they travel to an academic medical center and spend days in a classroom. At its worst, the education comes at the wrong time, in the wrong place, from the wrong individual.

If a family doctor sees an odd skin lesion on a patient—as in Dr. Koop's story of Joe's freckle—that doctor cannot then wait six months to sit in a classroom or library to find out what it is and how to treat it. In his own locale, there may be no way of researching the problem, since the physician may not have access to a research library. A small clinic would be an unlikely repository for the latest medical literature. Using the telemedicine network, which eliminates the need for journals on the shelf, the rural doctor can download to a computer whatever medical information is required from the centrally located data bank at MCG. Complemented by a telemedicine consultation, the network, in effect, allows for "just-in-time learning."

The system, of course, can also be used for a more standard configuration of medical education. Doctors at the various remote sites can gather around their monitors to attend lectures instead of driving all the way to a university hospital. And with telemedicine extending the specialists' ability to see what is going on outside the high walls of their hospital, that lecture is likely to have greater relevance.

Through this multi-media tool, students can be introduced to human physiology, nutrition information and disease prevention. MCG's interactive health care program is linked to 110 primary and secondary education "distance learning" classrooms, with the aim of bringing preventative medicine to the classroom and episodic care to students attended by a school nurse. It will, as Sanders says, "help us teach our kids about smoking, AIDS and popcorn." Hopefully, the network will eventually help eliminate the problem of delayed and inappropriate care that affects so many schoolchildren.

In many schools, even in affluent areas, if a child gets sick during the day, he or she is sent home. Since it is often the case that both parents are at work, the pediatrician's office is closed by the time a child's parents get home. The mother and father must then bring the child to the emergency room of a hospital—the wrong place, from a medical and economic perspective, to care for a fairly simple health care need.

Finally, a robust telemedicine network enhances continuity of care. It can avert the physical and mental stress of having an extended hospital stay in a city far from home. In fact, as MCG has demonstrated, the patient may not even have to leave home. The home-based system described in the first chapter has practically all the functionality of the hospital-based system. Most likely, a similar model for monitoring patients in the home can be used for nursing homes and related facilities.

Telemedicine's network is the future of health care—in surgery, at home, in education and elsewhere.

11

Hospital 2000

The health trade is characterized by a rapid development of medical technology. This applies to advanced instruments for diagnosing and treatment, drugs, technical remedies for nursing and biotechnology. One of the greatest challenges for the health services is to match the expectation of the population to the services which can be delivered on a large scale.

J. Nymo
Telektronikk, January 1993

Steve DiNapoli has a brain tumor. His surgery is scheduled for 8:00 A.M., so he arrives at the hospital the afternoon before. Handing his meditag to the admissions clerk, he watches her insert it into a desktop computer. A summary of Steve's medical history, address and other identification information flows from the clerk's personal computer into the hospital's central database. A minute later, the clerk returns the tag to him and says, "You're checked in, Mr. Smith. Before you go upstairs, would you like to store any valuables in the safe?"

"No thanks," he says, wondering if he'll need any valuables after this is over.

When Steve goes upstairs, the supervising nurse puts his tag into another computer to extract the latest magnetic resonance images (MRIs) of the tumor area and other data needed for the surgery. The nurse takes a pen from his pocket and touches a block on the computer screen:

"I've just sent your pictures to Dr. Dodd, Steve." He then writes a quick message on the screen and touches the pen to another block to transmit it:

"I've just paged him so he knows you're ready to be briefed on the surgery."

Dr. Dodd tells Steve about the upcoming surgical experience, from anesthesia to possible outcomes. After recording pre-operative notes on a pocket-sized computer that recognizes handwriting and speech, Dr. Dodd goes into his office to design and practice the delicate operation. To begin, he wirelessly transmits his new notes from the hand-held computer to the full patient record on his desktop computer, aiming and pushing a button as easily as if he were changing television channels with a remote control. The note on line eleven was an order for a specific post-operative medication. He underlines it on the screen with his electronic pen, then touches a little block that says "Rx." Instantly, the order is transmitted to the hospital pharmacy.

Dodd then reviews other elements of Steve's record, which include a videotape of a three-way telemedicine consultation involving Dr. Martin, an oncologist in Paris; Steve's family doctor in Texas and himself in New York. In addition, a sketch created by Dr. Martin and annotated electronically, shows a possible surgical route to the tumor. Combining the latest MRI images with stored data about the anatomy of the surgical region, Dodd maps out the operation on a computer generated, three-dimensional simulation. The image of Steve's brain has photo-realistic quality.

Furthermore, in the virtual-reality environment that Dodd creates to map out and rehearse his surgery, objects "know" how to behave. It's a process called behavioral modeling that allows the "virtual brain" and the "virtual tumor" to have the same physical characteristics as the real things. Since Steve's brain has a tumor within it, it no longer has the same characteristics as a "normal" brain. Dodd therefore has to program such changes as consistency and location of surrounding tissue into the model.

The next day, Steve is wheeled into the operating room (OR) of the future. Given the spectrum of the surgeon's informational needs and the technology available to meet them, this OR cannot be just an updated version of our nineteenth century model. It features a surgical workstation, the conduit for multiple types of patient-specific images, auditory and text data; the location from which telepresence surgery is initiated; the control panel for robotics activity and the site where surgical simulation occurs.

To make the leap from the nineteenth century to the twenty-first, creative teams of medical and design experts will use virtual reality to produce an innovative design for the operating room of the future. In the "virtual environments" they create, all the contributors to the design process will be able to freely move tables, television monitors, lights, cables, robots and other elements into place. The movements of people, the role of shadows, the cost of equipment—all of these factors will have already been analyzed.

The teams "move" things in and out of the virtual space with two of the standard tools of virtual reality—a helmet with miniature television screens mounted in front of the eyes and an instrumented glove, called a DataGlove by its developers at VPL Research. The surround-view helmet conveys a sense of being inside a room. As the wearer looks up, the ceiling is visible; looking left reveals an open door leading to another room or some other configuration.

The glove is a so-called gesture-input device. In ordinary computer systems, the typical input device is a keyboard; in some it's a pen or voice. However, while wearing the DataGlove, the wearer's movements command the computer to act precisely.

Made of smooth Lycra, the glove has fiber optic cables, or flex-sensors, that run along the back of the thumb and fingers. On the back of the hand sits a one-inch cube—a sensor that helps establish the hand's place in space. The sensor ensures that the hand moves where the user wants it to move within the virtual environment. The optic cable goes down to the tip of the finger and thumb, makes a circle and comes back. The system emits a beam of light and measures the time it takes to go to the hand and back. Bending the hand creates more reflections, so it takes longer for the light to go from the beginning, around the loop, to the tip of the finger and back. That's how the system measures the amount of flexion in the fingers.

At the same time, the cube on the back of the hand, or magnetic tracker, projects in which direction the hand is pointing. Working together, all these sensors tell the system where and when the operator's hand grasps, moves forward, twists or releases a tool. The visual effect seen in the helmet is the operator's disconnected hand, or hands, grasping objects, moving them into place, holding instruments and discarding unwanted items. This same technique is used in surgical simulation.

This seemingly fantastic operating room of the future will still contain some of the old technology, but in a more multi-functional way than its predecessor. As a surgical facility at the hub of a telemedicine network, it can receive and transmit patient data used by physicians at both the operative site and the site of the patient's continuing care. The MRIs, images from the digital microscope and vital sign information gathered on the spot can shape the surgery and be integrated with a video tape of the procedure in a teaching file. The OR of the future is, overall, a place equipped for curing, training and even conducting research. It is also a place where traditional problems of the surgical environment can be overcome through software, equipment redundancy, placement, design and more. These "traditional problems," which had caused device failures, mishaps with lasers and electrocautery accidents, can instantly negate all the skill a surgical team has.

Luckily for Steve DiNapoli, some of these futuristic techniques have already been tested and are being used today. As Steve's operation begins, Dr. Dodd superimposes a three-dimensional MRI image over the patient's head. The tumor is defined in bright green, while the healthy tissue surrounding the malignancy is deep blue. This, in effect, gives the surgeon "X-ray vision." Without this visual assistance, it is highly likely that the tumor's boundaries would be uncertain and healthy tissue—and perhaps bodily function—could be needlessly lost forever.

This particular surgery requires extraordinary precision. Dr. Dodd elects to use telepresence. In preparation, he programmed the telepresence system with the map he developed on his surgical simulator the previous evening. In concert, then, with the enhanced visual acuity afforded by the MRI superimposition, the surgeon has defined limits of movement on the system. Healthy tissue cannot be invaded by the robotic arm unless the surgeon overrides his own programming. The surgeon's own muscle tremors, no matter how small, are filtered out at the surgical workstation a few yards away from the operating table.

Reaching into the next generation of telepresence, difficult and delicate surgeries will no doubt be performed by intelligent robots preprogrammed by the world's most talented surgeons. Other than program design, the physician who designed the operation may have no actual involvement in the surgical procedure.

The new surgical techniques used in the OR of the future will require special training beyond that which is now taught in medical schools whose students practice on cadavers and animals. Innovations such as the ability to have X-ray vision, to control tremors or to map out operations in advance, will expand and nurture surgical skills in new realms. Surgical simulation using virtual reality technologies will help practicing specialists as well as residents sharpen their skills. This will ensure that the high-technology helps lead to better outcomes for patients, whether they are on an operating table in the same room as their surgeon, or three thousand miles away.

Col. Rick Satava, the doctor who heads efforts in hardware innovations at the Advanced Research Projects Agency, also funds some of the civilian efforts to design and build the operating room of the future. He feels that surgery is finally on the verge of a radical departure from the nineteenth century model, largely because of digital technology:

> There is finally a realization that medicine may actually be a small subset of "information with a medical flavor." Everything we need to know about a patient can be brought to the surgeon in electronic (digital) form, such as video images during surgery or teleconsultation, CAT or MRI scans, laboratory data, medical record and vital signs. . . . the surgeon can now palpate, manipulate and even operate by moving joysticks or surgical handles that send electronic signals to instruments that do the task. Thus the key to the future is the digital physician who brings information into the monitor of a surgical workstation and can act by sending electronic signals to the remote site. In essence, we can dissolve time and space.

In a separate wing of the hospital is a room that has some similarity to the operating room of the future, but it is a world away from the talk of tumors and trauma. Equipped for virtual-reality simulation, high-speed data collection and transmission and closed-loop therapies, the big difference in this space—the delivery room of the future—is that the patient is usually awake, noisy and happy to be there.

The roles of virtual reality in the delivery room of the future include pain control, monitoring labor and coaching the prospective mother through the birthing process. As a pain reliever, virtual reality provides a vivid, three-dimensional distraction during hours of labor. One woman may choose to drift into a beach resort; another may want to animate the subtleties of the birthing process. As a tool for the obstetrician, a virtual reality system keeps the doctor precisely informed of the progress, or any abnormal movements, of the baby in the birth canal. Finally, the virtual-reality simulation serves as a birthing coach. The mother sees, in real-time, what effect her breathing, shifts in position and "pushing" have on the delivery. It's a way of getting it right the first time, instead of going through the trial and error that generally makes a second or third birth easier.

Sometimes the birthing process is much more abrupt. A baby could be born severely premature, with lungs so underdeveloped that it cannot breath air. In the delivery room of the future sits a special "trauma pod" for the infant—a liquid-filled incubator. Inside, chemicals called perflurocarbons carry oxygen to the tiny collapsed lungs as the baby breaths comfortably, just as it did for many months in the liquid-filled womb. Decades ago, before the pioneering work of Leland Clark, Jr. in liquid breathing technologies, perflurocarbons were just a by-product of America's nuclear research.

The monitors, simulators and incubators in the delivery room of the future not only reduce stress and fear for the mother, but for the obstetricians, as well. With a 78 percent chance of being sued for malpractice, an obstetrician in the United States needs every advantage possible in ensuring the safe delivery of a child. There is also a strong possibility that the devices aiding in future deliveries will radically reduce the number of caesarean sections. This procedure now takes place in one-quarter of all American deliveries—and about one-third are unnecessary. In the United States, a caesarean section boosts the delivery bill by roughly $4,000.

Strange though it may seem, this leap forward for the medical community owes part of its evolution to the electronic gaming industry and Hollywood. Science fiction for children of all ages has popularized virtual reality to the extent that the technology of make-believe, three-dimensional worlds has become more affordable in the medical environment. For example, a Silicon Graphics central processing unit and high-resolution monitor cost a quarter of a million dollars before the dinosaur movie, "Jurassic Park," was made. A year later, that same technology cost less than half the price of the original. Those who think that it's a horrible waste of ingenuity to put virtual reality games into arcades and other entertainment venues should consider the plethora of benefits this kind of mass popularity has brought to medicine.

As a training medium, virtual reality can help put to rest the old adage "Physicians bury their mistakes." Instead of a fledgling surgeon performing surgery on live patients under the watchful eyes of a professor, the new and future doctor can practice on virtual organs until he or she gets the procedure right.

There are different ways to use virtual reality as a training device. Many seem to have been lifted from a futuristic Hollywood movie script. For example, in the virtual environment, the surgeon preparing for gall bladder surgery sits at a workstation. She puts on a surround-view helmet and DataGloves. The image in the helmet is of the internal organs of the lower abdominal area. When the surgeon decides to cut, she opens her hand and—just as if it were an operating room—says, "Scalpel." An assistant sitting at a keyboard hits the key that means scalpel and it appears in the surgeon's virtual "hand." Through the use of voice input technology, it is possible to eliminate the need for a surgical assistant by directly asking the computer for an instrument. The hands in the virtual environment work together to perform the incision, retract, snip and extract. When the surgeon wants to discard an instrument, she opens her hand quickly and simply flicks it away. High technology, keen anatomic knowledge and procedural accuracy make the experience seem real.

Another new approach, used in eye surgery simulation, is the kind being pioneered by researchers at the Georgia

Institute of Technology and the Medical College of Georgia. In this simulation, the surgeon begins in the conventional fashion—by sitting down in front of a microscope. The microscope is attached to a Silicon Graphics workstation, however. Surgical tools used in the simulation provide the same kind of force feedback that makes telepresence surgery seem so real. The tactile sense of cutting, combined with the sight of blood and layers of the eyeball, train the surgeon in a no-risk environment.

These streamlined tools of virtual reality will also help a patient at home. Steve's operation went flawlessly, but what if the operation had left him with some impediments? His motor skills would be temporarily diminished and his ability to speak impaired. Rehabilitation would be needed. During the early stages of healing, Steve would practice manipulating the fingers of a DataGlove to signal a computer that synthesizes speech. This use of the DataGlove also has applications in telemedicine for non-speaking patients who want to communicate with a doctor long-distance.

Another of the innovative devices which can interface with virtual reality devices is the DataSuit, a tool for measuring human motion. Using a DataSuit during exercise, our patient Steve could send precise data on his progress to the physical therapist, whether he was still at the hospital or at home. Greenleaf Medical Systems of Palo Alto, California, which develops computer-based medical technology for clinical diagnosis and therapeutic intervention, is pioneering applications of the DataSuit in health care.

Unlike the DataGlove, which is a one-size-fits-all device that can be easily recalibrated for each individual, the DataSuit is a customized body suit. Both the suit and glove collect data dynamically in three-dimensional space. Sensors track the full range of motion as a person bends, twists, grabs, punches or waves. This fresh capability offers a broad range of possibilities for diagnosis, remote or on-site, as well as continuing monitoring and rehabilitation in the home or other sites away from specialists.

Beyond far-reaching home therapy and rehabilitation, applications for the DataSuit include areas like sports medicine and training and repetitive strain injury prevention. The ingenious suit will be capable of helping athletes learn better ways of coping with injuries and improving performance. Other uses could include designing equipment or work processes to prevent types of repeated stress injuries like carpal tunnel syndrome, an affliction suffered by many data entry workers.

Cutting-edge treatments can be aimed at potentially fatal illnesses as well as other serious conditions. Some operations, like hip replacements and root canals, must be done over and over again today because the ability to correct the condition the first time is limited by the surgeon's eyesight and muscle control. As Robodoc illustrated, new technology can avert the need for revisions in hip replacements by boring a hole so precise that no cement needs to be added to fill the gap between a real bone and an implant.

Examples of the technology of the telemedicine revolution are also reaching dentistry. The setup of a small camera and microscope, similar to that in the MCG telemedicine system, is used by Dr. Joseph Grenn, a faculty member at the Pacific Endodontic Research Foundation, to do root canals. Whatever he sees in the microscope is displayed on a television screen above the operative site. At the same time he presses the compound into the canal—like pushing a tight cork into a wine bottle—his assistant sees it on the screen and knows which instrument the dentist needs.

Brain surgery may be more dramatic, but breakthroughs in dentistry will probably have more widespread appeal. The microsurgical procedures pioneered at the La Jolla, California Foundation, by founder Dr. Gary Carr and his faculty, give patients unprecedented assurance that they only have to endure the procedure once.

The breakthroughs expected in the next generation of procedures have a common theme emerging: the surgeon will be able to view things clearly that would once have been partially or totally obscured. New applications of imaging technology such as MRIs, creative configurations of existing technologies such as the scope-and-camera setup, and breakthrough technology such as virtual-reality workstations will radically change what happens everyday in hospitals around the world.

12

Prevention 2000

It is difficult, even hazardous, to attempt to describe a scientific breakthrough while it is still in progress. . . . Nevertheless, there occasionally is a scientific breakthrough of such overwhelming implications for society that its importance is immediately recognized.

Jerry E. Bishop and Michael Waldholz
Genome

Global monitoring, via the various communication modes used in telemedicine, will be part of the needed technology for disease prevention in the future. Generations to come will talk about infectious disease and inherited disorders in a purely historical sense. As our world shrinks because of modern commerce and transportation, there will be a new and somewhat frightening recognition that diseases we thought eradicated are actually still rampant in other areas of the world.

For instance, malaria, all but eliminated in America and Western Europe, is still the world's greatest single killer infection. When a mosquito bites, it injects a culture of parasitic cells into the victim's bloodstream. As if running for their lives, the parasites race to the liver. They multiply, grow and reenter the blood to invade the red blood cells. At the present time, the pharmaceuticals industry has mefloquine, chloroquine or pyrimethamine to keep the parasites at bay, but such drugs don't work in all cases—especially as new viral and bacterial strains continue to appear. The biosciences industry has great hope for a new combatant—taxol, extracted from the Pacific yew tree. Better yet would be a technology which can eradicate the mosquitoes' existence before they threaten an entire village or town.

Because many new areas of telemedicine technology are arising, not only diseases but other serious problems can be solved. Remote sensing, another technology of telemedicine, has a role in disease prevention that places it squarely in the digital revolution. NASA, for instance, has used satellite pictures to spot aberrant crop conditions for decades. The information flow provided to other countries has been steady and useful in early detection of agricultural problems.

The principles are similar to those applied to human disease. There are specific environmental determinants that affect the presence and abundance of threats to health, such as mosquitoes that cause malaria or sleeping sickness or ticks that cause Lyme's disease. With the technology provided by telemedicine, remote sensors are able to identify and measure changes to those determinants, finally giving scientists a dependable way of predicting the occurrence of serious problems. In the case of a mosquito, the environmental determinants include rainfall and terrain. Within the regions that have the right topography, there are specific types of vegetation that serve as the larval habitat. The remote sensors actually measure visible light and infrared emissions. In this context, particular attention is paid to the reds and greens, which portray differences in vegetation. The computer then takes the reflectance data and interprets it, thus making it possible to predict and eradicate areas where disease will be.

Studies recently conducted by the Uniformed Services University of the Health and Sciences combined remotely sensed information about environmental and vegetation changes with mapping technology. They demonstrated with nearly perfect accuracy the ability to distinguish which villages—even which houses—in the test sites were at high risk for malaria. Instead of wasting their limited public health funds on spraying everywhere, the Mexican government could immediately target problem areas.

Global telemedicine will permit, a dedicated medical satellite equipped with remote sensors to generate its own data, but would also receive data from the other locations on earth which are part of the disease control ground operation. This data would be incorporated into the satellite's geographic information system. The results would then be sent to a primary site for quick analysis by a supercomputer and bounced back up to the communication satellite. The satellite would then relay the information back to ground stations so that formerly uncontrollable epidemics and serious conditions could be routinely handled.

On a smaller scale, the Mayo Clinic's experimental use of NASA's new digital satellite technology also illustrates telemedicine's potential in disease prevention. When the Mayo Clinic first tried to apply the Advanced Communication Technology Satellite (ACTS) technology to telemedicine, it reached out to Native Americans at the Pine Ridge reservation in South Dakota. Located on the southwestern border of the state, Pine Ridge is one of the most economically underdeveloped areas in the United States. Of the nearly 25,000 people who reside on the reservation, less than half have running water, less than one-third have telephones and 80 percent of personal income comes from welfare. Because health care is so scarce, many people endure chronic illness, particularly diabetes. In fact, Native Americans suffer from the world's highest rate of lifestyle-induced diabetes. Fetal alcohol syndrome is a common culprit, attacking young minds and bodies.

To compound the problem, Indian Health Service in the United States enforces strict limitations on referrals to facilities outside the reservation. Usually, a transfer happens only in critical or life-threatening situations. In many cases, this becomes a hideous example of bureaucracy and racism, systematically killing people who could recover with the right treatments.

Once aware of this horrendous situation, Mayo officials decided to put the ACTS workstation at Pine Ridge after exposure to the seriously defective logic affecting health care on the reservation. Among the individuals seeking help was a twenty-one-year-old man who had a dermatological problem so serious that open sores covered his entire body. The cause had not been determined, and ointments did little to relieve his constant pain. Although treatment at Mayo offered the prospect of a cure, the man could not get a referral to go off the reservation for medical care because his was not a life-threatening condition.

At Pine Ridge, not only individuals but the group as a whole also suffers. For instance, leaders within the reservation had fought for four years to get an ultrasound machine. Finally, the government released the money for it. In a situation rife with cruel humor, however, the government did not release any funds to train the resident technician in how to use it.

At places like Pine Ridge, a telemedicine network cannot change the environmental factors that nurture lifestyle diabetes or fetal alcohol syndrome. However, utilizing telemedicine's techniques and innovations can lead to disease control and prevention. Because telemedicine can treat symptoms remotely, doctors can document and investigate patterns of illnesses, commonalities between cases and attitudes of patients. Such abilities will make health education available in ways never before tried and thus meet the needs of Pine Ridge's residents. Hopefully, it will equip the broader medical community with a greater ability to avert the same problems in other places where adequate medical care was never before offered or even possible.

The strongest hope for preventing a great number of diseases, including alcoholism and certain forms of diabetes, lies in genetic engineering. Telemedicine, in providing a link for the great scientific minds of the medical research world, can expedite the curing of many mysterious diseases. For example, one type of diabetes, the onset of which has nothing to do with lifestyle, is called "familial nephrogenic insipidus" (FNDI). People affected by it have a constant raging thirst matched by the urge to urinate. They pass gallons of urine a day and drink gallons of water to keep up with the urinary dehydration.

Specialists from around the world pooled their research to track down the genetic culprit. At first, they observed that a majority of the FNDI patients were male. Males have only one X chromosome, therefore FNDI was blamed on a single mutant gene located on the X chromosome. Researchers thought this was the "vasopressin receptor" gene because they found it mutated in the FNDI patients they studied. They also thought it was a recessive trait.

Dr. Eltan Friedman, an endocrinologist who is currently researching the disorder, theorized that less than one-hundred families throughout the world might carry the defective gene. Top researchers were able to reach these families on a personal basis by using the technology of telemedicine. Among them are descendants of Scottish people who landed in Nova Scotia in 1761, four families in Sweden, three in Israel, two in Brazil and nine in the United States. Obviously, unlocking the door to the genetic secrets of this disease had to be a very focused effort.

One Brazilian family who was contacted by the researchers helped them find clues which contradicted previous theories, however. Spanning five generations, the Brazilian family had twenty-one of its seventy-eight members afflicted with FNDI. This gave evidence that there was a dominant rather than recessive mode of genetic transmission. There was also no evidence of a mutated vasopressin gene. Finally, they learned that more than half the victims were actually female.

In mid-1994, after more telemedicine-aided international searching, Friedman came up with a new theory: the corrupt gene is a neighbor of vasopressin's that has to do with the processing of water in the kidney. If he's right, then the next step is correcting the genetic defect by gene therapy.

Telemedicine's ability to enable scientists to track down and personally communicate with remotely located patients, or families having a history of a particular disease in areas of the world where there are few doctors or few specializing in that disease, is a major breakthrough in the future of health care.

13

Litigation 2000

In medicine, the efficacy of a new development must be balanced with the potential for harm. This idea is stated succinctly in the classic ethics admonition, "Do no harm." . . . But telemedicine, as a system of health care delivery, like its face-to-face counterpart, suggests little possibility of harm. Rather, harm seems more likely to occur from its non-use.

Jane Preston, MD
The Telemedicine Handbook

In the modern marriage between humans and machines, there can be many impediments. Healthcare of the new frontier means doctors in routine collaboration with computers, robots, imaging devices and electronic communicators. Some of these have already begun, others will begin soon. In hundreds of instances so far, orthopedic surgeons have worked side by side with robotic hip replacement specialists. In brain surgeries, previously inoperable tumors are being removed because magnetic resonance imaging (MRI) gives surgeons X-ray vision.

But hardware can fail: a wayward gurney can break a surgeon's leg; a loose screw in a robot can render it unstable; a camera lens can crack. Software problems are even less manageable and harder to rectify.

On the positive side, a confluence of intelligence and complex programming in human beings and machines yields sources of new hope for patients. On the negative side, the more complex the programming, the less likely it is that it will ever be debugged or made flawless. Nothing's perfect. Something will go wrong someday. From a legal point of view, it is just a question of who, or what, will be responsible for the damage.

At the first Mayo Clinic Telemedicine Symposium, Dr. Collins and Dr. Charboneau speculated on what could, on a bad day, have happened to their liver tumor patient whose surgery had been so successful. What if the specialist in Arizona had failed under his colleague's remote guidance instead of saving the patient's life? In their endeavor to understand the pros and cons of telemedicine, they scripted the following negative version of the satellite consultation as follows:

Bill: "Joe, I'm not seeing the location of the needle as well now as I was a few minutes ago."

Joe: "Yeah, I'm having trouble seeing it also."

Bill: "Joe, I hope you can see where you are because I can't."

Joe: "Bill, he's having some chest pain, which I think is angina. We're giving him nitroglycerine now. I think we're going to have to hurry this along."

Bill: "Right. I understand, but I still can't see your needle."

Joe: "The needle is out now."

Bill: "Where is the alcohol?"

Joe: "The alcohol is in. I got as close as I could."

Bill: "Uh-oh. That doesn't sound good!"
Joe: "Bill, he's having a lot of chest pain now. I'm going to have to sign off and take care of things here. I'll call you later and let you know how it all turns out."
Bill: "Right. Good luck."
THE FOLLOWING DAY:
Joe: "Bill, it's been a really bad twenty-four hours. This whole procedure turned into a complete disaster. The good news is that our patient is still alive. But he's in intensive care. He is in a lot of pain. We just got his CAT scan, which shows a large area of bleeding next to the tumor. I feel terrible. The family is very upset."
Bill: "This sounds awful."
Joe: "The family has also been asking a lot of questions about how we did this."
Bill: "What do you mean?"
Joe: "I told them I had discussed the case with one of our doctors in Rochester who had experience with the procedure and that you were watching over the satellite to make sure things turned out well. It turns out that the patient's son-in-law is a lawyer and he intends to hold us both responsible."
Bill: "You've got to be kidding! I don't even have an Arizona medical license."
Joe: "Yeah, that fact came up in the conversation with the son-in-law. He really got upset then."
Bill: "But I've never even been to Arizona!"
Joe: "I have been talking with our Legal Department. I think there's probably going to be a lawsuit coming out of this."
Bill: "Oh, no!"
Joe: "Maybe you should be talking with Mayo's lawyer in Rochester."

Bill: "I can't believe this. I wish I'd never gotten into this teleradiology stuff. How can *I* be held responsible for consulting on a case that *you* did a thousand miles away?"

If the act of a single surgeon were to lead to a bad outcome, an accusing finger could be pointed at one individual. If a needle broke during the procedure, and that product failure caused the problem, the accused could be the needle manufacturer. In this case, there are two doctors, two technicians, several cameras and satellites, an encryption device, cables and a needle involved. Telemedicine vastly expands the number of people and businesses legally vulnerable in one case.

On one hand, it could be argued that interactive television gives the physician an unusually good way to manage risk—video tape everything and store the tape as a visual record. The presence of a complete audio and video record of a consultation, combined with the use of electronic instruments with enhanced diagnostic capability, could be a doctor's dream come true. Jay Sanders at the Medical College of Georgia definitely thinks so:

> For the first time, we're opening up the communication modality as a potential source of misinformation. It's fascinating nobody has brought this up before relative to the telephone. You call the doctor and he says, "Take two aspirin and I'll see you in the morning"—that's never been challenged. . . . But think about the fact that we now not only have a written record, we have a visual record, we have an audio record of the entire consultation. We think that's being aggressively defensive in terms of malpractice.

In fact, it is often a lack of good records that leaves medical professionals open to attack in a malpractice suit.

Bernard L. Crowe looks at the situation another way. As

head of the Health Technology Division for Australia's Institute of Health and Welfare, he has explored issues holding back the development of telemedicine in Australia. All these extra images, he has speculated, "could result in an increase in litigation once patients realize that such information is readily available."

The possibility of technological innovation creating new legal soft spots is enough to alienate some physicians. Some will resist the use of telemedicine technology as long as possible. It is easy to understand why. In the United States, for example, the average physician has a 37 percent chance of being sued at some time in his or her career. This increases to 52 percent for a surgeon and 78 percent for obstetricians. A Harvard University study confirmed what doctors have long suspected: a physician's chance of being sued for medical liability bears little relation to whether he or she has been negligent. In fact, 80 percent of the studied claims filed for medical negligence studied did not even involve a negligent adverse effect.

The possible legal tangles of utilizing telemedicine may make physicians liability status even more precarious. For instance, remember Steve DiNapoli whose brain surgery was discussed in an earlier chapter? If Steve's surgery—performed in the world of telemedicine—had gone awry, his physician might have new concerns about the consequences of using high-technology innovations. Virtual-reality assisted telepresence surgery could lead to an even greater legal conundrum.

First of all, virtual reality is a lie. In other words, virtual-reality applications are simply models of real things, and as such, they are abstractions. "Irrelevant" elements of the real environment, or real anatomy, are filtered out in order to create a vivid, sensually gratifying illusion. So, while the end result may be convincing and immensely useful, it is not exactly the same as the actual subject.

Other things can go wrong as well. Human error could sabotage the precision of the robot. An instrument of the wrong size in the hands of an innocent robot might cut too deeply. Would the technician or nurse who put it at the operative site be responsible for the negative surgical outcome, or would the doctor who remotely picked up the instrument be at fault? Or would the company that made the robot be liable because it should have been calibrated more precisely? Or maybe it would be the fault of the hospital administrator who should have known better than to buy imperfect robots and hire careless people?

Who gets sued in the practice of telemedicine, as well as the relative chances of winning a case, has everything to do with the availability and integrity of the electronic evidence. In today's world, a paper record can be misfiled, tea-stained, ink-smeared, reduced to unclear print on a photocopier or ripped. Maybe it's because paper has been in use for so long, but people generally seem more tolerant if the marred, unreadable or misplaced file is on paper than if it is a computer record. Electronic data storage is supposed to be better. Usually it is, but there are numerous variances that make some electronic files better than others.

The issue of image and audio quality sparks a range of reactions from practitioners who use telemedicine systems. For cost reasons, telemedicine and medical image storage systems commonly rely on data compression. It is another approach to eliminating "irrelevant" information. Compression technology squeezes the information into a smaller package by throwing away all data unnecessary to delivering an image or sound of acceptable quality. For example, video is sent frame by frame, with each frame corresponding to a still picture. Each succeeding picture changes as motion progresses. Bits of data unchanged between frames are not transmitted with each frame. The compression process, therefore, means selecting only the elements within a video signal that must be transmitted with each frame to maintain an accurate image. Then, using mathematical algorithms, the computer minimizes the amount of data needed to represent this information.

In telemedical application, compression has not presented any known negative outcomes. Nevertheless, the Mayo Clinic maintains that loss is unacceptable in a specialist environment, where physicians consult on a much more detailed level. Dr. Bijoy K. Khandheria, a cardiovascular disease specialist at Mayo, is an outspoken critic of data compression in many medical areas:

> What if I look at an image and I say I don't have any doubt, and send the patient away? The first thousand [times] I may be right. It's patient one thousand and one where I may be wrong.

Patient records might also contain images and sound that were enhanced for diagnostic purposes. The mammograms created with the direct digital imaging system can involve computer processing to make calcifications more evident. Film X-rays can be digitized then processed to improve image quality. The electronic stethoscope vivisects the sound of a beating heart. Would the enhanced images and the altered sound that led to diagnoses be admissible in court as original data? Out of the many images comprising each case, would the courts attempt to determine which computer-enhanced version should have been used for diagnosis in order to prove the guilt or innocence of a doctor?

In some places, these questions are still meaningless. Some courts will not yet admit computer records as evidence. Standards for managing them are just evolving. In litigation, one of the first things in question is whether or not the records are complete. Patient charts in the paper-based world reflect what the health care provider chooses to write or draw. Once it is done, however, it is generally respected as a "permanent" record. In the electronic world, this would logically translate into keeping all the videotapes and images generated in all telemedicine consultations.

At some point, keeping all these records could become a storage problem, even though storage technologies are also advancing rapidly. Could one or both physicians on a case agree that elements of the video and audio record are irrelevant and edit them out, or would that be considered illegal tampering with a patient's record? Unless the medical and legal communities, nationally and internationally, arrive at some protocols for computer recordkeeping, there will be some strange but important legal and practical challenges for care-givers in the telemedicine arena.

The scenario of the failed tumor ablation, as shown by Dr. Collins and Dr. Charboneau at the beginning of this chapter, brings up another facet of the liability issue. When a telemedicine network is used to enhance patient care across a state or country's border, is the distant doctor practicing outside the territory that accepts his or her medical credentials liable? This is an issue which impacts the international medical community.

In the United States, for instance, physicians are licensed on a state-by-state basis, except in the military health care system. While it can be argued that the patient is "transported" electronically to the doctor, which is what would have happened in the physical sense before telemedicine, the reverse has also been argued. The out-of-state consulting physician, because he or she is affecting care in another jurisdiction, would be perceived by some to be practicing illegally. In view of all kinds of modern highways, whether made out of asphalt or fiber optics, the state-by-state, country by country licensing system is truly antiquated. It is also illogical, considering that physicians take national examinations for board certification and licensure. Bypassing the issue by gathering multiple licenses is expensive and time-consuming, with doctors potentially spending tens of thousands of dollars on annual renewal fees. On an even more practical, patient-centered level, the existing licensing structure could inhibit disaster assistance through telemedicine consultations. The push toward a national licensure, and international agreements, will undoubtedly grow stronger as telemedicine programs proliferate.

In the past, the automobile heralded an era of personal mobility. The personal computer signaled immense opportunities for productivity. Now, the technology of telemedicine offers real prospects for more innovative and personalized medicine.

As more and more people partook of modern luxuries, conveniences and higher standards of living and working, items and conditions which were part of these conveniences came under scrutiny. When cars failed structurally or the smell of carbon monoxide made people sick, the automobile became the symbol of a selfish, destructive society. When office workers began suffering from carpal tunnel syndrome from long hours at keyboards, and pregnant data entry clerks felt they miscarried because of electronic emissions, the once welcomed computer gained the image of being the tool of heartless, greedy businesses. It can only be expected that the machines of telemedicine, and those who make and use them, will have many image—and legal—problems, too, as both the assets and deficits of the utilization of new complex technologies in health care become more widespread.

14

Ethical and Privacy Issues

The "clipper chip"—aptly named, as it clips the wings of individual liberty—would encode for [United States] Federal perusal whenever a judge rubber-stamped a warrant, everything we say on a phone, everything we write on a computer . . . Add to that stack of intimate data the medical information derived from the national "health security card." Combine it with the travel, shopping and credit data available from all our plastic cards, along with psychological and student test scores. Throw in the confidential tax returns, sealed divorce proceedings, raw files and CIA dossiers available to the Feds, and you have the individual citizen standing naked to the nosy bureaucrat.

William Safire
Essayist

The script of medical progress has leading roles for new types of villains, as well as heroes. Unlike the doctor, technician or product manufacturer who might inadvertently cause a bad outcome for a patient, there are those who *choose* to do harm.

Just as telemedicine vastly expands the number of people and businesses legally vulnerable in one case, so does it expand the number who are potentially unethical. Though there are many technological and human safeguards that can be put in place to protect patients' rights to privacy and confidentiality, there are some things in the world of telemedicine which cannot be guaranteed.

In the realm of biotechnology, knowing one's genetic secrets will not be as private as remembering one's dreams or nightmares. For example, if you have a genetic susceptibility to alcoholism, your employer might gain access to this usually private information and deny you a promotion. If you are planning to deliver a baby who has cystic fibrosis, your insurer or health care provider may know this information. If your genetic map points to Alzheimer's, your potential spouse who gains the knowledge of it may decide he or she cannot deal with the difficulties the disease would present in the future.

Digital technology is advancing at an unbelievable rate and the benefits of this technology in telemedicine are miraculous. But with any new technology there are drawbacks that have to be addressed as well. For example, while on the way to Zagreb, Croatia, to deploy a portable telemedicine system, two Army doctors stopped by a fountain in Landstuhl, Germany. One of them carried the system's digital camera. He photographed his colleague sitting on the stone border around the fountain. Shortly after that, he also photographed a voluptuous young German woman near the same spot. Later that day, he downloaded both photos into a computer, then started to toy with the images.

Digital images are essentially a collection of dots. The stone of the fountain might be varying shades of gray and brown dots with the doctor's shirt in green dots. If the doctor does not look good in green, certain computer applications make it easy to change the dots to orange, or to change the pattern of his shirt to stripes. If only a picture of the fountain is desired, the man can be removed.

As a joke, the doctor who took the digital photos inserted the image of the young woman into the picture with his friend. Anyone looking at the retouched version, including a wife or girlfriend, would have thought twice about the man's innocence. After the laughter stopped, the perpetrator destroyed the file in the computer. It was a potent demonstration to the telemedicine team of how easily digital records can be manipulated if they fall into the wrong hands. If the photographer had an evil motive, he could have just as easily sent the photo, electronically or printed, to the man's wife or to a newspaper.

Electronic transmission of patient records is supposed to be a confidential process—direct from one health care provider to another. The combination of encryption technology, which severely limits access to computer files, and a high standard of ethics should wrap the data in a tight web of security. It is not impossible or improbable, however, that someone inside or outside a hospital could electronically intervene, capture the record and alter it. This unscrupulous person could then sell the information to someone in the media willing to print it.

Encryption technology can range from relatively affordable coders-decoders (codecs) to systems designed for spies. On the high end is the "B/MAC" (Type B/Multi-plex Analog Component), which scrambles the signal on the transmission end and descrambles it on the receiving end. Used by the Mayo Clinic, B/MAC separates color from black and white, audio from video, and digitizes everything. Then, by using random codes, it embeds the audio into the video and sends it as individual lines that are scrambled. Each picture line is moved around the picture and reassembled at the other end. The computer code changes the lines about every 1/60 of a second, so it is virtually impossible to steal the signal. In technology, though, what is impossible today often becomes routine tomorrow.

Computer databases can provide automatic security by limiting access and prohibiting duplication. For example, using the technology of intelligence gathering agencies, a multi-user secure database may allow Nurse A to enter on one level of security, whereas Doctor B would enter at higher level. Even different physicians might have different levels of clearance for a particular database. If one person with access to a patient's records attempted to add or change something, the system could be programmed to do a number of things: not accept the changes, alert the system manager when the change was made and what it was, redate the file and so on. Again, this is based on spy technology, so it is still uncommon in the hospital environment. In an ideal world, the technological barriers to tampering would be high. In truth, the best protection costs the most, so medical records of royalty, presidents and movie stars will probably be more secure than those of ordinary people.

A broader view of the situation relates to the ethical aspects of access to costly types of diagnosis and treatment. In characterizing his country's approach to universal health care, Norwegian Birger Nymo wrote in *Telektronikk* that it is "based on the principle of treatment on the lowest efficient level of care." This is not to say that Norway does not aspire to higher levels, but that the nation has a practical standard for giving everyone access to health care. In that situation, it could be a long time before cutting-edge technologies move into routine use. In the United States, for instance, there is no policy of universal access, but average people who can get to the Mayo Clinic, for example, can have the benefits of current research and high-end medical technology.

Average citizens who are ill generally rely on government to enforce their rights as patients. It is not clear whether many countries, provinces and states are prepared to do this, however, in a high-technology medical environment. Even in the current, paper-based system, confusion reigns. In the United States, for example, each individual state has laws that cover the creation, authentication, storage, editing and discarding of medical records. It is the same situation with laws protecting a patient's privacy or the disclosure of health-related information. Information that is safe and private in Lausanne, Switzerland may go unprotected in Los Angles, California. When computers are part of the scheme, part of protecting patients' rights means defining what an electronic "original" is, the role of computerized signatures to authenticate records and how much information has to be stored.

In the area of biotechnology, ethical considerations involve some very complicated issues of genetic privacy, screening for genetic disorders, access to research data or materials and human subject research. Genetic information is now commonly used by prospective parents to make decisions about getting pregnant or carrying a fetus to term. Aggressive testing of Jewish people, particularly those of Eastern European origin, for Tay-Sachs carrier status has dramatically reduced the number of children who suffer from the disease. Tay-Sachs first causes paralysis then kills the child, usually by age five. Before the test for carrier status was developed, only a prenatal screening would reveal the problem—no help for parents unwilling to consider an abortion.

An example of the hidden dangers of testing for genetic diseases is the case of Ann and John. Ann and John want to have another baby, but their first child was born with cystic fibrosis. When Ann becomes pregnant again, she decides to be among the 750,000 people this year in the United States to request prenatal testing for the condition. The test indicates that the fetus is also afflicted with the condition. Because their first child has only a very mild form of it, they decide to take their chances and have the baby. The insurance company, because of the enormous costs of having a child with cystic fibrosis, send them a letter saying that the couple has a choice of aborting the fetus or losing health care coverage.

Ethical considerations often bridge over to financial ones, and can go down two different roads. The new technologies can reduce costs related to health care, or be a new source of profit. Both are powerful forces. Neither is inherently good or bad.

Health care, from the perspective of whoever or whatever is paying for it, is not free. The positive side of genetic testing is the possible discovery of information that could help someone avert the onset of coronary artery disease, thereby reducing medical bills. The negative side comes with the discovery of information that could mark a person as "high risk," a potential source of expense for an employer or insurer. From an employer's perspective, business could suffer by hiring a "defective" person. Knowing that Candidate A for a vice-presidency has a genetic susceptibility to coronary artery disease, whereas Candidate B does not, could mean no job for Candidate A.

Biotechnology miracles, such as the kind that help desperate women get pregnant, highlight the profit potential of medical breakthroughs. Egg donations, as dangerous and painful as they can be, earn healthy fees for the donor and those who extract the eggs. Post-menopausal women in their fifties and sixties in several countries have become biological mothers after embryo transplants. Market forces clearly drive the research and therapy enabling this phenomenon. Research using fetal tissue and embryos could also be a mechanism for profit. In the extreme, that means that abortions could become a part-time job.

To counter the prospect that profit incentives will override societal welfare, Canada's Royal Commission on New Reproductive Technologies has advanced a proposal for national and international consideration. This proposal recommends that genetic and reproductive technologies be guided by social policy, not market forces. To achieve this goal, governments should form and empower citizen-run groups to establish guidelines on how biotechnology should be used.

One possibility is that doctors engaging in genetic and reproductive research and therapies would be licensed for a set time only. Periodic review of the work to assure compliance with the established guidelines would be required. It would also be clear that fetal tissue donors would be just that—donors. No payment would be allowed. As for the wealthy sixty-year-old woman who wants to have a baby, that's an issue that exposes multiple layers of debate on children's rights. For one, if the egg used were donated, could the child later become the victim of a dispute over which "biological mother" is better able to provide care?

Medical technology is forging way ahead of laws regarding the rights of patients and society. Some of the same advances that are making telemedicine possible are also opening up a "brave new world" of moral and legal conundrums. In the rapidly changing medical environment, a culture of compliance with ethical behavior and a code of professional standards of conduct are our main sources of comfort

15

Space Age Infrastructure

Life and death in technology is a matter not of revenues but of prospects. Vacuum tubes reached a pinnacle of sales in the seventies. Revenues from telephones and televisions are currently at an all-time peak. But the industries organized around these two machines will not survive the century. Still, telecommunication executives want to believe that televisions and telephones can evolve bit by bit into the new digital world. . . . This dream cannot come true. Even to talk of "telephones" and "televisions" reflects a lexicographic lag. . . . In the coming years, the very words will ring as quaintly as "horseless carriage," "icebox," or "picture radio," today.

George Gilder
"The Death of Telephony"
The Economist

In the world of telemedicine, a new, inventive vocabulary has emerged which enables communication between those bringing about Digital Age technology. The language goes along with sweeping concepts like "personal communication" and "global connectivity." These concepts describe the practical application of advances in communications and computations—advances that are bringing the telemedicine revolution to life.

The concept of "digital" is leading to a massive discussion within the context of telemedicine. Some of that discussion is critical to understanding the nature of the new information changing health care. Everyday, this information is flowing to and from telepresence surgical systems, smart cards, trauma pods, video equipment and other tools of the revolution. Knowing the way information flows is also fundamental to making long-distance medical magic become more realistic and achievable.

Of course, the projection of these exciting, sweeping concepts to their future potential involves more complex ones. Today, most telemedicine systems use a combination of video, still images and different kinds of audio data to provide consultative, diagnostic and educational services to patients in remote areas.

The pictures and sound may be picked up and transmitted as analog (continuous) signals, or as digital (discrete) signals. If a picture being shown is analog, there is theoretically no end to the number of subtle changes in the image. For example, the color gray in the analog world is an infinite number of shades moving from black to white, or vice versa. If the picture is digital, it's made up of dots, or pixels. In a high-resolution, digitized image there are 256 steps of gray. To the human eye, however, there still seems to be no end to the number of subtle changes in the image.

The reason such specialized leaders in areas of the telemedicine field at the Mayo Clinic rely on an analog system is its ability to capture the exact nature of the original image and sound and send it to another site. Since Mayo's primary telemedicine activity has been in specialty medicine, physicians at the clinic want the assurance that every hue, every line, every shape, remains intact when they share information.

In contrast, most other telemedicine systems transmit digital signals. One of the reasons is cost. Transmitting a digital signal can be done much less expensively than sending an analog one.

In an interactive video consultation or videoconference, the eye perceives things in real time if the picture is transmitted at a rate of thirty frames per second. In digital expression, this is roughly ninety million bits (discrete parts) of data per second. Standard phone lines don't handle this kind of transmission. If they did, it would take well over a million phone lines working together to send a single picture in real time.

Bundling the lines creates a more powerful conduit. Coaxial cable, the technology used to send television channels into homes, is a cable designed to handle more traffic than phone lines can. Capacity ebbs as distance increases, so cable systems include amplifiers that periodically boost their strength. Now, technology allowing this cable to be used for high-speed multimedia data networking gives it a greater value in the telemedicine network. Cable carries about six times the the traffic of T1 lines and costs less.

A broadband Integrated Services Digital Network (B-ISDN) line is an all-digital telephone line that can simultaneously handle large quantities of data, voice and video. Fiber optic cable can transmit at the rate of 1.3 billion bits per second, and the more efficient 2.7 billion bps fiber should soon become readily available. In Tokyo, where the government is considering a $900 billion investment to build a comprehensive telecommunications network, experts are experimenting with transmission rates of ten billion bps. In short, these are the options for a terrestrially-based telemedicine network.

Unfortunately, populations in rural and remote areas that most need modern medicine's innovations are not near anything more sophisticated than standard phone line technology, if that. Jim Reid, founding director of the Eastern Montana Telemedicine Project, says, "The infrastructure development in rural areas is about twenty years behind the times." Estimates on when fiber optics will finally come to rural and frontier areas of the United States, for instance, run from ten to twenty years. The options for reaching these places with real-time interactive video are extremely limited and expensive. For example, due to various tariffs governing communications in the United States, it is more expensive to use land lines between the Mayo Clinic in Minnesota and a town in a neighboring state than it is to do the same thing between the Clinic and its Arizona counterpart over twelve hundred miles away.

Wireless communication options are microwave, cellular and other applications of the radio spectrum. In an earthbound microwave system, signals that are powerful enough to handle real-time video are transmitted from one point, or tower, to another. The downside of microwave use is that signals may be degraded by atmospheric disturbances like rain or fog, or environmental obstacles such as walls. Finally, there is the earth-sky microwave system, or satellite. As the world has seen the Olympics and Academy Awards coverage, satellites offer the bandwidth to deliver real-time image transmission. However, the use charges are daunting for most health care facilities. This is another major obstacle that emerging satellite technology must surmount or find a substitute for.

In the case of the Mayo Clinic, because of its unique requirements, elected to set up a full-motion video system that does not use compression technology. Compression entails transmitting images in a shorter period of time. The essence is that if it takes one second to send one thousand pieces of information, it will only take one-half second if that data can be represented in five hundred pieces of information. The bandwidth needed for this is enormous; satellite transmission was the only option, considering the distances between sites. While satellite transmission has inherent advantages in terms of image quality, it also raises concerns over privacy and cost. Encryption technology and serendipity dissolved these concerns.

The original system's cost came to around $5 million, including consulting, construction, installation, purchasing satellite dishes, shipping and other associated expenses. At the time, the high cost was compounded by transmission fees of $375 per hour, paid to GTE Corporation, for leased satellite time. Mayo's planners had anticipated needing twelve to fifteen hundred hours per year. This small amount did not warrant much of a price break. By 1991, when they responded to increased administrative and medical use of the system by adding a second channel, transmission costs were exorbitant.

Meanwhile, GTE's new satellite, GStar III, was having its own difficulties. After being ferried by a shuttle, a failure in one of its motors caused it to slump into a useless orbit. In terms of its commercial value, it became space junk. Scientists at the company then configured a design that would put it close to a geostationary orbit. It combined the effects of the satellite's thrusters with the gravitational pull of the earth. A year later, after using up a significant amount of fuel, GTE logged a dubious success. The satellite was usable again, but still not in a stable orbit near the equator. GTE cut a deal with Mayo that gave the company a tax break and the clinic a solution to its soaring costs: free tracking equipment and an enormous discount on the transponders that would lock into the wandering satellite. At a standard cost of at least $10 million per transponder, getting three for $4 million had great appeal. Mayo accepted the deal and, as a result, turned a positive cash flow by February 1994. Thus, prior to the purchase, Mayo made up what was spent on the transponders as compared to what would have been spent leasing time as an occasional user. Now, transmissions are essentially free to the Clinic until the satellite disappears, sometime in 1997.

Among the most innovative of the emerging transmission technologies is one called the Advanced Communication Technology Satellite (ACTS). This is the first all-digital satellite that NASA has built. Whereas other satellites have one beam that covers the country, ACTS demonstrates spot-beam technology with smaller beams of about two hundred miles in diameter that overlap. Through high-speed on-board switching, ACTS can pick up data from one beam and send it off to another. This offers at least three interlocked advantages. First, because it is beam technology, the power is concentrated in a smaller spot, resulting in high data throughput with a smaller antenna on the ground. In short, 600 million bits per second can be achieved with a three-meter antenna, not, as before, with twenty-meter antenna. The design also gives ACTS store-and-forward capacity.

Another benefit of the design is that use charges can be tied directly to how many seconds or minutes it takes for the beam to grab the data and take it away. In that sense, it's more like a phone system. In contrast, lease charges on standard satellites reflect hourly rates. First designed in 1985, ACTS was not launched until late 1993 because of funding snags stemming from the Challenger disaster. The satellite embodies, therefore, some "old" thinking about transmission modalities, even though it still represents new possibilities. While its usefulness in areas equipped with fiber optic cable is questionable, ACTS can make a significant difference to areas that won't see optical fiber for a long time.

For telemedicine, this important discovery allows an increased capacity to concurrently send transmissions that require a lot of bandwidth. For example, because of the technological breakthrough, a formerly unthinkable scenario could take place. Jay Weinbaum, a patient, is critically ill with a cardiovascular problem. A top cardiologist in New York has been asked to do an emergency consultation. ACTS, angiograms, echocardiograms, electrocardiograms (EKGs) and other high-resolution images could be sent quickly while the specialist listens remotely to the patient's heart and consulted with the primary care physician. Further commercial prospects, cost and efficiency will be determined in the future after the Mayo Clinic completes telemedicine experiments using ACTS. In the meantime, NASA has issued licenses to the ACTS technology so that commercial ventures can get underway.

Solving another major problem, Low Earth Orbiting Satellites (LEOS) could offer a feasible solution to the problem of reaching remote areas. They could also transform satellite communication into a real-time experience because of imperceptible delays between transmission time and signal receipt. A low-earth orbiting satellite sits in an orbit about six hundred miles above the earth. Conventional satellites rest in a 22,300-mile orbit, having a very noticeable signal delay of about one second.

With the LEOS project already in place, the satellite Satellife now features a network called HealthNet that is used for intercontinental consultation between physicians. Memorial University of Newfoundland, home of the longest continually operating telemedicine program in the world, serves as the North American terrestrial interconnection point, or gateway, for Satellife. Motorola's Iridium project plans to place a constellation of sixty-six LEOS in space by 1998. In its first generation, the Iridium satellite would simply be devoted to telephony, offering global voice, fax, paging and data transmission services, but not full-motion video. X-rays, EKGs or other medical images could be sent over the system, which would have a store-and-forward capacity. Concentrating on making the technology cost efficient, Motorola expects the cost of sending a compressed X-ray of acceptable quality to cost between $15 and $50. In contrast, it cost the U.S. Army an average of $80 to send a compressed X-ray from Somalia to Walter Reed Army Medical Center over the Inmarsat system.

Of course, what are inexpensive costs to some organizations and countries are to others impossible to bear. While many nations of the world cannot afford to bring land lines to the people in remote areas who need communications most, LEOS could meet their voice and data transmission needs quickly and affordably. In some parts of Africa and South East Asia, there are up to eighteen thousand people per doctor. Telemedicine will bring them some reasonable heath care options for the first time.

There is a possible drawback of both the Iridium and Teledisc schemes, in that roughly seven thousand pieces of space debris threaten the performance of the three hundred or so satellites already in a high orbit. In this regard, Microsoft Corporation mogul Bill Gates has effected a joint venture, known as Teledisc, with McCaw Cellular. He has proposed blanketing the sky with over two hundred low-orbit satellites, which would handle a broad scope of services and expand the telemedical applications for LEOS.

Telemedicine networks may involve both wired and wireless modalities, thus they will face many of the same problems as national and international corporations do. They would have to lease set amounts of satellite time, or lease dedicated land lines at a fixed cost per month, in order to send their data. Standards such as asynchronous transfer mode (ATM) have emerged to solve the problem with "bandwidth on demand," which is a pay-as-you-go approach to getting whatever transmission capacity is required. ATM, developed for high speed data transfer, breaks voice and data information into chunks, or tiny cells of equal size. Cells are pushed through the network and reassembled so quickly that callers or computers do not detect any gap between them. ATM is a way of putting various transmission modalities to work more efficiently. Widespread use is anticipated and could certainly make the difference between a cost-effective, even profitable, telemedicine network and a financial loser. The cells are like standardized shipping containers, with the customer paying only for the "space" occupied by their information, rather than the whole method transportation

Solving these technical issues is fundamental to the

future of health care, as is finding the answers to the ethical, moral and legal dilemmas raised by technology's advancements. People who need distant medical expertise will obviously be out of luck if there is no electronic path leading to their door. Their situation won't be any better, however, if they are linked to a system which ignores high standards of health care delivery and a clear policy of responsibility to the patient.

Conclusion

Unleash your hope. That is the strongest message from emerging medical technology. As citizens of the Digital Age, we can laugh at old movies in which giant metal men and mutant tomatoes attacked small children. Research in robotics and genetics instead makes once-unimaginable surgeries routine and deadly diseases avoidable.

Tools of the telemedicine revolution are improving the odds for patients in multiple ways. Computers and communications devices have moved health care toward time and distance independence. A corollary process is the transformation of health care delivery systems from doctor-centered to patient-centered, and that means more personalized diagnosis and treatment. Finally, medical practitioners can access real-time continuing medical education instead of advice after mistakes are made. All this and the sun, moon and stars, too?

In a way, yes. The same technology that helps doctors reach remote earthquake victims and battlefield casualties projects their expertise into space. An electronic house call on the space station Mir is not much different from one to a distant Russian village.

And yet, in this promising future, there could be a house of horrors. Technology of the telemedicine revolution could inspire unwelcome phenomena. Machines can break; fears of a robot on "autopilot" slicing too far through an abdominal wall could become reality. Somebody will violate the rules; use of genetic test results in screening job applicants could cause an abuse of critical breakthroughs in preventative medicine. Genius can destroy as easily as it can build. Cracking the code protecting medical data transmissions might be a game to a student or electronic media aficionado, but not to those whose private parts end up on a strange person's computer screen. Patients could become so fearful of distant medical care that they refuse it.

Of course, we must find ways to avoid, or at least mitigate, these potential horrors so mankind can focus on the stunning benefits of new technology. For example, medical professionals could halt a patient's fear of technology before it ever takes hold. In the context of an interactive television consultation, Dr. James Brick, a founder of Mountaineer Doctor Television in West Virginia, says very simply to his colleagues:

> You've got to spend some time with the patients when you get on [television] with them. Socialize with them at the beginning. I don't think you can stress this enough. We all learned this when we were in medical school. If you go in to talk to somebody, you have to get to know them.

Dr. Brick, Dr. Jay Sanders, Dr. Max House and other telemedicine leaders are helping the world take the revolution one step at a time. On the horizon are a multitude of ideas and plans, some fantastic and some realistic, to offer telepresence surgery for brain tumors and virtual reality simulations. In the meantime, today's practical, cost-controlled telemedicine systems highlight the benefits of integrating communications and computing technology into health care in a way that make these innovations seem warm—more an extension of human caring than an experiment or novelty.

As a guiding principle for the explorers who are pushing back the frontiers of medicine, "Do no harm" cannot guide the pioneers of the telemedicine revolution. "Do more good" comes closer to what should be said. These researchers and doctors are risk-takers—not with their patients, of course, but with their careers and goals. Nebulous or conflicting laws addressing digital devices in a medical environment, and equipment that requires special training to use are just two serious concerns. Impediments such as these serve as deterrents to taking a leadership role in telemedicine and other applications of modern technology in medicine.

Doctors who do take this role must be ambassadors and communicators who have higher aims. They must be willing to share their expertise over a global network, often for no compensation. Canada, Norway and the United States are just three of the nations with thriving telemedicine networks where doctors have little or no financial incentive to extend their networks to other, less advanced countries. Rather, their only incentives are visions of a better health care future.

Then again, there are some doctors who keep themselves out of the telemedicine revolution because they think it is ridiculous to invest in technology when more "fundamental" supplies are scarce. When the United States Army's portable, and relatively cheap, telemedicine system was bridging the gap between Zagreb, Croatia and Walter Reed Army Medical Center in Washington, D.C., one disgruntled Army doctor commented to the press back home, "We need tongue depressors and they're buying computers." In addition to basic medical supplies, he clearly lacked both vision and a cost-benefit analysis.

It is true that the cost of an innovation like the experimental digital mammography machine or ROBODOC can run $250,000. It is also true that identifying the gene linked to cystic fibrosis costs about $150 million. Most advanced research projects to find answers to the complex diseases, and most of the medical care which must be provided in our modern world, is costly. But not as costly in terms of human life as the status quo. How can hope be unleashed if access to the necessary technology or further research will be seriously restricted by cost?

As Dr. Jane Preston has said—to her colleagues worldwide, to the United States Congress and to health agencies—health care needs a whole new economic model. For many patients in distant places around the world, who would otherwise die or become disabled, telemedicine could be their salvation. It could mean no lost wages, no temporary housing for family members, no repeated diagnostic tests and no shocking bills from a big-city hospital. Breakthroughs in robotics and microsurgery mean far fewer serious operations like hip replacements and root canals, because the needed surgery can be done correctly the first time. Genetic mapping and other biotechnology ventures can mean prevention of and cures for diseases that can attack people through decades of fear and degeneration. Finally, other innovations equip people who cannot move, speak or see with the ability to express themselves. These are not tools that, for now, save money, but those that enable. They can change the forecast of people who might not have hope. The cost of technology and biotechnology research should not be judged superficially, but in the long term—in the children and adults saved who can then contribute to our civilization.

The wondrous outcomes that can be created by competent medical professionals with new technology have been described as miracles. If they were just incomprehensible feats, however, there would be very little reason to unleash our hope for a healthier future. Fortunately, they aren't miracles at all. They are instead demonstrations of the human race's unlimited creativity and its capacity to build a better world.

appendix 1

Selected Programs Worldwide

Australia

Children's Hospital at Westmead, Sydney, New South Wales:
a teleradiology system designed to provide pediatric diagnostic services nationally and internationally

Canada

Memorial University Health Sciences Center, Newfoundland:
the oldest continually running telemedicine program in the world

France

Hôpital de Bicètre, Université Paris:
a telemedicine system focused on enhanced pathology services

International Space University, Strasbourg:
site of the central campus of a world organization for training and academic instruction in all areas relating to space, including space life sciences

Germany

Immunomedics Inc., Dusseldorf:
conducting clinical trials of cancer imaging devices that identify tumor sites

Japan

Kyoto Prefectural University of Medicine, Tokyo:
the only site in the world that has used high definition television in health care delivery

Norway

University Hospital of Tromsø:
serves Norway's scattered population in the northern half of the country

Russia

Star City, Moscow:
linked with Johnson Space Center in Houston, Texas in preparation for cooperative efforts to Space Station Mir

MedTel Cominform, Moscow:
developing portable satellite transceivers in hope of creating a network of short "spacebridges" throughout Russia

Singapore

Telecommunication Authority:
installing advanced communications systems throughout the island to facilitate a wide range of information services, including telemedicine

Switzerland

Swiss Federal Institute of Technology, Lausanne:
pioneering work in instrumentation and robotics for surgery, including innovations in spine surgery and biopsy procedures

United States

Walter Reed Army Medical Center, District of Columbia:
portable telemedicine systems for the battlefield use (Remote Clinical Communications System) and a teleradiology program using direct digital imaging, or filmless X-rays (Medical Diagnostic Imaging Support)

Medical College of Georgia, Augusta:
a statewide, multi-functional program, with a pilot program to put telemedicine in the home

Kansas University Medical Center, Kansas City:
special focus on teleoncology services, and documentation of the impact on rural cancer patients

Uniformed Services University of the Health Sciences, Bethesda, Maryland:
the site of key research in the area of telepathology, including the efforts to use remote sensing to improve health conditions around the world

Massachusetts General Hospital, Boston:
in collaboration with Harvard University on several projects, including a telemedicine trial involving broadband transmissions and project to design the operating room of the future

The Mayo Clinic, Rochester, Minnesota:
expanding services to the Indian Reservation at Pine Ridge, South Dakota; host of international telemedicine symposia

Dartmouth Hitchcock Medical Center, Hanover, New Hampshire:
researching applications of virtual reality and other emerging technologies; home of the C. Everett Koop Institute

Brown University, Providence, Rhode Island:
maintains a satellite link with the Russian Space Research Institute (IKI) that is used to exchange data, including U.S. space mission information

LDS Hospital, Salt Lake City, Utah:
pioneer in closed-loop systems (that is, a signal on the patient's condition goes to a computer, the computer makes a decision about therapy, then institutes the therapy)

University of Washington School of Medicine:
designing a computerized model of the human body using detailed images of actual human parts recorded in digital format; will result in a massive database of images that can be rotated to any angle, magnified and manipulated; plans to offer services through the Internet

appendix 2

How to Build a Telemedicine System

Alleging there is something like a turnkey telemedicine system to deliver long-distance health care draws criticism from medical professionals. The fact remains that certain elements are shared among robust systems worldwide. Following is a technical overview of the Medical College of Georgia network, which serves as a good example of a workable system configured primarily from commercially available, "off-the-shelf," technology. (Note: Approximate 1994 prices are included parenthetically to establish cost relationships.)

Camera One ($2,000) is for patient interviews. This "meet and greet" camera is just standard videoconferencing equipment that provides about half the resolution of broadcast quality video.

Camera Two ($8,000), or the main diagnostic camera, has 16-power zoom, tilt and pan capabilty. The quality of the signal is much higher than Camera One, the quality of the color balance is higher, and the realism associated with the image is much better. The 16-power zoom capability is contingent on the lens aperture settings. The more expensive the camera and lens set, the more likely it is going to allow for greater resolution, and less distortion, of the magnified image. It sits on a swivel mount ($1,500).

Camera Three ($3,000) has lenses allowing for tremendous resolution, especially at a close range. Considered the "document camera," this one-chip unit is capable in some instances of substituting for the main diagnostic unit.

Camera Four ($2,700), the microsoakable camera, went through a couple revisions to be as useful as it currently is in telediagnosis. The camera was not designed for telemedicine systems, but for laparoscopic procedures. A hand-tooled adaptor connects it to the full range of scopes used in eye, ear, intestinal, cell and other examinations. Unlike the earliest attemps at adaptation, the current model provides an auto-focusing function to virtually eliminate discomfort for the patient.

For purposes of using the first camera, the patient interview camera, there is interactive compressed video. (Any time a diagnostic image is sent, it is a one-way transmission, which implies a reduced requirement for compression.) The codec (coder-decoder, $27,000) accomplishing the compression enables a choice of network interfaces, from low-cost, dial-up, switched services to dedicated networks. It has special ports for peripherals, built-in encryption for transmission security, and automatic conversion from United States television standard (NTSC), to the the European (PAL). The Communications Standards Package ($8,500) covers international modes.

The Video Image Capture Board ($1,800) is the "frame grabber," or tool for accomplishing freeze-frame video.

The control system relies on a touch panel, or screen ($3,400).

The audio system is high-end, including a digitizer/encoder ($2,500) and wireless microphone system ($2,000).

The package would be essentially complete with the addition of a VCR, monitor, power supply, modem, video routers and peripherals.

When added together, all of the hub hardware costs about $100,000; the cost for a the remote-site set-up is closer to $120,000. The cost of signal transmission varies greatly from state to state, nation to nation, depending on the availability of ordinary phone lines, fiber optics, satellites time and so on.

Selected References

Anselmo, Don. "The Iridium Project, Global Communications and Access to Care in the Third World." Presented at the Mayo Telemedicine Symposium, October 2, 1993.

Bashshur, Rashid; Patricia Armstrong. "Telemedicine: A New Mode for the Delivery of Health Care," *Inquiry*, Volume XIII, No. 3. September 1976.

Bird, Kenneth T.; Rashid Bashshur; et al. "Telemedicine: Concept and Practice," *Telemedicine: Explorations in the Use of Telecommunications in Health Care*, 1973.

Billica, Roger D., MD; Charles R. Doarn. "A Health Maintenance Facility for Space Station Freedom," *Cutis*, Volume 48, October 1991.

Bishop, Jerry E.; Michael Waldholz. *Genome*. Touchstone, New York, NY, 1990.

Collins, Joseph M., MD; William Charboneau, MD. "Long Distance Procedures: Legal, Licensing and Reimbursement Issues."

Presented at the Mayo Telemedicine Symposium, October 1, 1993.

Desai, A.B.; et al. "Telemedicine—A Feasibility Experiment for National Application," *Indian Pediatrics*, Volume 21, October 1984.

Doarn, Charles; Donald Stewart, MD; Joseph Dervay, MD. "Spacebridge to Moscow: Formally Kicked Off." *CommonHealth*, December 1993/January 1994.

Eger, John M. "A New Agenda for Health Care in the New Millennium: The Role of Telecommunications." Presented at the Mayo Telemedicine Symposium, October 1, 1993.

Gilbert, Francoise. "Telemedicine: Using Computer and Telecommunications Technology in the Delivery of Healthcare—Selected Legal Issues," draft of June 1994.

Gomez, Lt. Col. Edward R., MD "Global Telemedicine—Impact on Operation Restore Hope." Presented at the Mayo Telemedicine Symposium, October 2, 1993.

Harris, Bernard A., Jr., MD. "Space Adaptation Syndrome and the Implications of Telemedicine." Presented at the Mayo Telemedicine Symposium, October 2, 1993.

House, A. Max, MD. "The Canadian Experience: Using Telemedicine for the Support of Medical Care at Remote Sites." Presented at the International Telemedicine/Disaster Medicine Conference, December 9-11, 1991.

______. "Distance Health Systems—Canadian Collaboration," Presented at the Mayo Telemedicine Symposium, October 1, 1993.

______. "Update on Telemedicine." A report of the

Memorial University of Newfoundland, 1993.

Houtchens, Bruce A., MD; et al."Telemedicine and International Disaster Response: Medical Consultation to Armenia and Russia Via a Telemedicine Spacebridge." Presented at the International Telemedicine/Disaster Medicine Conference, December 9-11, 1991.

______."Telemedicine and International Disaster Response," *Prehospital and Disaster Medicine*, Volume 8, No. 1, January-March 1993.

Jones, Mary Gardiner. "Electronic House Calls: 21st Century Healthcare Services for Consumers." Presented at the Mayo Telemedicine Symposium, October 1, 1993.

Levy, Alden B. "DataGlove & DataSuit in Medical Applications of Virtural Reality." Prepared for the IMAGE Society Conference, June 17, 1994.

Lindberg, Donald A.B., MD. Testimony; National Institutes of Health, May 2, 1994.

Miner, Nadine E. "Using Voice Input & Audio Feedback to Enhance the Reality of a Virtual Experience." Presented at the IMAGE Society Conference, June 17, 1994.

Nymo, B. J. "Telemedicine," *Telektronikk*, January 1993.

O'Neill, John J.; Joseph T. Nocerino; Philip Walcoff. *Benefits and Problems of Seven Exploratory Telemedicine Projects*. For the Department of Health, Education and Welfare Public Health Service, February 1975.

Park, Ben. *An Introduction to Telemedicine*. The Alternate Media Center at New York University, School of the Arts, 1974.

Preston, Jane, MD. *The Telemedicine Handbook.* Published by the Telemedical Interactive Consultative Services, Inc., Austin, Texas, 1993.

______; Frank W. Brown; Bette Hartley. "Using Telemedicine to Improve Health Care in Distant Areas," *Hospital and Community Psychiatry*, Volume 43, No.1, January 1992.

Reid, James. "Telemedicine in Montana, Will It Happen?" Presented at the Mayo Telemedicine Symposium, October 2, 1993.

Rheingold, Howard. *Virtual Reality.* Touchstone, New York, NY, 1991.

Rosen, Joseph, MD. "The Role of Telemedicine & Telepresence in Reducing Health Care Costs." Presented at the IMAGE Society Conference, June 17, 1994.

Rotondo, G. "L'Attualita: Evoluzione ed applicazioni recenti della telematica in medicna," *Minerva Medica*, Volume 77, January 1986.

Sanders, Jay H., MD "The 'Star Trek' Healthcare System." Presented at the Mayo Telemedicine Symposium, October 1, 1993.

______; Francis J. Tedesco, MD. "Telemedicine: Bringing Medical Care to Isolated Communities," *Journal of the Medical Association of Georgia*, May 1993.

Satava, Richard M., MD "Dual Use: Military & Civilian Use Medical Applications," Presented at the IMAGE Society Conference, June 17, 1994.

______. "High Tech Surgery: Speculation on Future Directions," *Minimally Invasive Surgery*. Edited by. John G. Hunter and Jonathan M. Sackier. McGraw Hill, 1992.

______; Stephen R. Ellis. "Human Interface Technology: An Essential Tool for the Modern Surgeon," *Surgical Endoscopy*, October 1993.

______. "Robotics, Telepresence and Virtual Reality: A Critical Analysis of the Future of Surgery," *Minimally Invasive Therapy*, 1992.

______. "Surgery 2001," *Surgical Endoscopy*, 1993.

______. "Virtual reality surgical simulator," *Surgical Endoscopy*, 1993.

______; I.B. Simon. "Teleoperation, Telerobotics, and Telepresence in Surgery," *Surgical Endoscopy*, 1993.

Stewart, Donald F, MD. "Medical Care Delivery in the U.S. Space Program," Presented at the International Telemedicine/Disaster Medicine Conference, December 9-11, 1991.

Tangalos, Eric G., MD. "Merging Tertiary Medicine with Telecommunications: The Mayo Clinic's Pioneering role in Telemedicine," White Paper, 1993.

Third U.S.-U.S.S.R. Joint Working Group on Space Biology and Medicine in Moscow and Kislovodsk, U.S.S.R. "U.S.-U.S.S.R. Telemedicine Consultation Spacebridge to Armenia and Ufa," Final Project Report. Presented at the December 1-9, 1989.

Watson, David S. "Telemedicine," *The Medical Journal of Australia*, Volume 151, July 17, 1989.

Index

C

D

E

F

J

K

L

M

Q

R

S

T